T0315572

INTERVENTIONAL CARDIOLOGY CLINICS

www.interventional.theclinics.com

Consulting Editor

MARVIN H. ENG

Transcatheter Mitral Valves

April 2024 • Volume 13 • Number 2

Editors

Marvin H. Eng
Firas Zahr

ELSEVIER

1600 John F. Kennedy Boulevard • Suite 1800 • Philadelphia, Pennsylvania, 19103-2899

http://www.theclinics.com

INTERVENTIONAL CARDIOLOGY CLINICS Volume 13, Number 2
April 2024 ISSN 2211-7458, ISBN-13: 978-0-443-13093-9

Editor: Joanna Gascoine
Developmental Editor: Akshay Samson

Interventional Cardiology Clinics (ISSN 2211-7458) is published quarterly by Elsevier Inc., 360 Park Avenue South, New York, NY 10010-1710. Months of issue are January, April, July, and October. Subscription prices are USD 224 per year for US individuals, USD 100 per year for US students, USD 224 per year for Canadian individuals, USD 100 per year for Canadian students, USD 317 per year for international individuals, and USD 150 per year for international students. For institutional access pricing please contact Customer Service via the contact information below. To receive student/resident rate, orders must be accompanied by name of affiliated institution, date of term, and the *signature* of program/residency coordinator on institution letterhead. Orders will be billed at individual rate until proof of status is received. Foreign air speed delivery is included in all *Clinics* subscription prices. All prices are subject to change without notice. **POSTMASTER:** Send address changes to *Interventional Cardiology Clinics*, Elsevier Health Sciences Division, Subscription Customer Service, 3251 Riverport Lane, Maryland Heights, MO 63043. **Customer Service: Telephone: 1-800-654-2452** (U.S. and Canada); **1-314-447-8871** (outside U.S. and Canada). **Fax: 1-314-447-8029. E-mail: journalscustomerservice-usa@elsevier.com (for print support); journalsonlinesupport-usa@elsevier.com (for online support).**

Reprints. For copies of 100 or more of articles in this publication, please contact the Commercial Reprints Department, Elsevier Inc., 360 Park Avenue South, New York, NY 10010-1710. Tel.: 212-633-3874; Fax: 212-633-3820; E-mail: reprints@elsevier.com.

CONTRIBUTORS

CONSULTING EDITOR

MARVIN H. ENG, MD
Structural Heart Program Medical Director,
Structural Heart Disease Fellowship Director,
Director of Cardiovascular Quality, Banner
University Medical Center, Phoenix, Arizona

EDITORS

MARVIN H. ENG, MD
Structural Heart Program Medical Director,
Structural Heart Disease Fellowship Director,
Director of Cardiovascular Quality, Banner
University Medical Center, Phoenix, Arizona

FIRAS ZAHR, MD
Associate Professor, Division of
Cardiovascular Medicine, Knight
Cardiovascular Institute, Oregon Health &
Science University, Portland, Oregon

AUTHORS

GHAYTH AL AWWA, MBBS
Cardiothoracic Surgery Fellow, Oregon Health
& Science University, Portland, Oregon

ABDULLAH K. AL QARAGHULI, MD
Research Volunteer, MedStar Health Research
Institute, MedStar Washington Hospital
Center, Washington DC

AHMED ALTIBI, MD
Fellow, Department of Cardiovascular Medicine,
Knight Cardiovascular Institute, Oregon Health
& Science University, Portland, Oregon

JASMINE ANJALI GARG, MD
Resident, Department of Medicine,
Westchester Medical Center, Valhalla, New
York

ANITA W. ASGAR, MD, MSc
Co-Director, Structural Heart Program,
Associate Professor of Medicine, Universite de
Montreal, Montreal Heart Institute, Montreal,
Canada

CHANDRALEKHA ASHANGARI, MD
Advanced Cardiac Imaging Fellow, Knight
Cardiovascular Institute, Oregon Health &
Science University, Portland, Oregon

VASILIS C. BABALIAROS, MD
Professor, Division of Cardiology, Emory
Structural Heart and Valve Center, Emory
University Hospital Midtown, Atlanta, Georgia

CARLA BOYLE, BSc
Medical Student, Division of Cardiology,
Knight Cardiovascular Institute, Oregon
Health & Science University, Portland, Oregon

SCOTT M. CHADDERDON, MD
Associate Professor, Knight Cardiovascular
Institute, Oregon Health & Science University,
Portland, Oregon

PRANAV CHANDRASHEKAR, MD
Fellow, Knight Cardiovascular Institute,
Oregon Health & Science University, Portland,
Oregon

CHANDAN DAS, MD
Cardiothoracic Surgery Fellow, Oregon Health
& Science University, Portland, Oregon

MARVIN H. ENG, MD
Medical Director, Structural Heart Program,
Division of Cardiology, Structural Heart
Fellowship Director, Director of
Cardiovascular Quality, Associate Professor of
Medicine, The University of Arizona, Banner
University Medical Center, Phoenix, Arizona

HAO KENITH FANG, MD
Chief, Division of Cardiac Surgery, Banner Universty Medical Center, Phoenix, Arizona

JASON R. FOERST, MD
Director, Structural and Interventional Cardiology, Virginia Tech Carilion School of Medicine and Carilion Clinic, Roanoke, Virginia

ANTONIO H. FRANGIEH, MD, MPH
Director, Structural Heart Program, Division of Cardiology, Associate Professor, Department of Medicine, University of California, Irvine, Orange, California

FADI GHRAIR, MD
Fellow, Structural and Interventional Cardiology, Virginia Tech Carilion School of Medicine and Carilion Clinic, Roanoke, Virginia

HARSH GOLWALA, MD
Assistant Professor, Department of Cardiovascular Medicine, Knight Cardiovascular Institute, Oregon Health & Science University, Portland, Oregon

ADAM B. GREENBAUM, MD
Associate Professor of Medicine and Co-director, Division of Cardiology, Emory Structural Heart and Valve Center, Emory University Hospital Midtown, Atlanta, Georgia

SAMIR R. KAPADIA, MD
Chairman, Department of Cardiovascular Medicine, Cleveland Clinic Foundation, Cleveland, Ohio

FARAJ KARGOLI, MD, MPH
Fellow, Division of Cardiology, Structural Heart Disease and Advanced Complex Interventions Fellow, The University of Arizona, Banner University Medical Center, Phoenix, Arizona

PATRICK S. KIETRSUNTHORN, MD
Fellow, Structural and Interventional Cardiology, Virginia Tech Carilion School of Medicine and Carilion Clinic, Roanoke, Virginia

JIN KYUNG KIM, MD, PhD
Professor, Division of Cardiology, Professor, Department of Medicine, University of California, Irvine, Orange, California

KRIS KUMAR, DO, MSc
Fellow, Oregon Health & Science University, Portland, Oregon

GURION LANTZ, MD
Assistant Professor of Cardiothoracic Surgery, Oregon Health & Science University, Portland, Oregon

CONRAD J. MACON, MD
Assistant Professor of Medicine, Division of Cardiology, Knight Cardiovascular Institute, Oregon Health & Science University, Portland, Oregon

JEFFREY A. MARBACH, MBBS, MS
Assistant Professor, Division of Cardiology, Knight Cardiovascular Institute, Oregon Health & Science University, Portland, Oregon

EMMANUEL L. MILLS, MD
TI Senior Clinical Research Coordinator, Knight Cardiovascular Institute, Oregon Health & Science University, Portland, Oregon

VINAYAK NAGARAJA, MBBS, MS, MMed (Clin Epi), FRACP
Interventional Cardiologist, Department of Cardiovascular Diseases, Mayo Clinic College of Medicine, Rochester, Minnesota

KHOA NGUYEN, MD
Cardiology Fellow, Division of Cardiology, Knight Cardiovascular Institute, Oregon Health & Science University, Portland, Oregon

POOJA PRASAD, MD
Fellow, Division of Cardiology, University of California, San Francisco, San Francisco, California

JAY RAMSAY, MD
Resident Physician, Department of Internal Medicine, University of California, Irvine, Orange, California

AARON R. SCHELEGLE, MD
Assistant Professor, Structural and Interventional Cardiology, Virginia Tech Carilion School of Medicine and Carilion Clinic, Roanoke, Virginia

TIMOTHY SIMPSON, PharmD, MD
Cardiologist, Oregon Health & Science University, Portland, Oregon

JOHANNES STEINER, MD
Associate Professor, Division of Cardiology,
Knight Cardiovascular Institute, Oregon
Health & Science University, Portland, Oregon

YICHENG TANG, MD
Cardiology Fellow, Division of Cardiology,
Department of Medicine, University of
California, Irvine, Orange, California

HIROKI A. UEYAMA, MD
Fellow, Division of Cardiology, Emory
Structural Heart and Valve Center, Emory
University Hospital Midtown, Atanta, Georgia

SALMAN ZAHID, MD
Fellow, Department of Cardiovascular
Medicine, Knight Cardiovascular Institute,
Oregon Health & Science University, Portland,
Oregon

FIRAS ZAHR, MD
Associate Professor, Division of
Cardiovascular Medicine, Knight
Cardiovascular Institute, Oregon Health
and Science, University, Portland,
Oregon

CONTENTS

Preface: Transcatheter Mitral Interventions: Multidisciplinary Progress at Its Best   **xiii**
Marvin H. Eng and Firas Zahr

Imaging of the Mitral Valve   **141**
Pranav Chandrashekar, Chandralekha Ashangari, and Scott M. Chadderdon

Echocardiographic imaging is the foundation for the evaluation of mitral valve dysfunction. Both transthoracic and transesophageal echocardiography provide insight into the anatomy, pathology, and classification mitral valve dysfunction. Echocardiography also provides a multi-parametric approach with semi-quantitative and quantitative parameters to assess the severity of mitral regurgitation and mitral stenosis. Transesophageal imaging is essential in the assessment of patients considered for surgical or transcatheter interventional strategies to treat mitral valve dysfunction. Cardiac computed tomography (CT) and cardiac MRI are useful adjunctive imaging techniques in mitral valve disease with CT providing detailed procedural specificity and MRI providing detailed ventricular and regurgitant flow analysis.

Mitral Transcatheter Edge-to-Edge Repair: Advancing Treatment Options for   **155**
Degenerative Mitral Regurgitation
Salman Zahid, Jasmine Anjali Garg, Ahmed Altibi, and Harsh Golwala

Degenerative mitral regurgitation (DMR) has earned great interest because of modern and innovative technologies emerging in its treatment. MR affects roughly one-tenth of those older adults over the age of 75. MR if untreated leads to adverse heart remodeling, resulting in left ventricular dysfunction, pulmonary hypertension, and heart failure syndrome. Despite surgical valve repair/replacement treatment being the standard of care, a significant proportion of severe MR patients face unmet clinical needs because of high or prohibitive surgical risks. This has led to the emergence of transcatheter therapies for high- and prohibitive-risk surgical patients, most notably mitral transcatheter edge-to-edge repair devices.

Functional Mitral Regurgitation: Patient Selection and Optimization   **167**
Pooja Prasad, Pranav Chandrashekar, Harsh Golwala, Conrad J. Macon, and
Johannes Steiner

Functional mitral regurgitation appears commonly among all heart failure phenotypes and can affect symptom burden and degree of maladaptive remodeling. Transcatheter mitral valve edge-to-edge repair therapies recently became an important part of the routine heart failure armamentarium for carefully selected and medically optimized candidates. Patient selection is considering heart failure staging, relevant comorbidities, as well as anatomic criteria. Indications and device platforms are currently expanding.

Functional Mitral Regurgitation: Transcatheter Therapy   183
Anita W. Asgar

Mitral regurgitation (MR) is one of the most prevalent types of valvular heart disease and is expected to increase in the next decade. Transcatheter therapies for MR are constantly being developed and studied for use in this population. In this review, the author describes the phenotypes of functional or secondary mitral regurgitation, discusses the potential therapeutic targets for transcatheter intervention, and reviews the results of such technology in the literature.

Mitral Regurgitation Complicated by Cardiogenic Shock: Reassessing Risk   191
Stratification and Therapeutic Strategies
Carla Boyle, Khoa Nguyen, Johannes Steiner, Conrad J. Macon, and
Jeffrey A. Marbach

Mitral regurgitation complicated by cardiogenic shock creates a unique and devastating risk profile for patients and poses significant difficulties for physicians who lack a comprehensive range of effective management strategies. Supportive measures such as intravenous vasodilators, intra-aortic balloon pumps, and percutaneous ventricular assist devices are often necessary to stabilize patients prior to definitive treatment with surgical mitral valve replacement or trans-catheter edge-to-edge repair. This review evaluates the evidence for the available supportive and definitive management strategies in patients with mitral regurgitation complicated by cardiogenic shock and presents a framework to aid clinicians in navigating the complex clinical decision-making process. Additionally, the authors review emerging transcatheter mitral valve replacement technologies that hold promise for expanding the therapeutic armamentarium and improving patient outcomes.

Postsurgical Transcatheter Mitral Valve Replacement   207
Faraj Kargoli, Abdullah K. Al Qaraghuli, Hao Kenith Fang, and Marvin H. Eng

Reintervention is commonly required postsurgical mitral valve replacement (SMVR) or repair due to bioprosthetic valve and annuloplasty ring degeneration. However, redo SMVR is associated with a high risk of morbidity and mortality. Postsurgical transcatheter mitral valve replacement (TMVR) is a safe and less-invasive alternative that has repeatedly been shown to be associated with improved survival and lower rates of complications compared with redo SMVR. Comprehensive patient evaluation and thorough procedural planning are key to successful TMVR.

Left Ventricular Outflow Tract Modification for Transcatheter Mitral Valve   217
Replacement
Hiroki A. Ueyama, Vasilis C. Babaliaros, and Adam B. Greenbaum

Left ventricular outflow tract (LVOT) obstruction is a life-threatening complication of transcatheter mitral valve replacement. In-depth analysis of pre-procedural computed tomography enables accurate prediction of this risk. Several techniques for LVOT modification, including Laceration of the Anterior Mitral leaflet to Prevent Outflow ObtructioN, preemptive alcohol septal ablation, preemptive radiofrequency ablation, and Septal Scoring Along the Midline Endocardium, have been described as effective strategies to mitigate this risk. This review aims to explore the indications, procedural steps, and outcomes associated with these LVOT modification techniques.

Orthotopic Transcatheter Mitral Valve Replacement   227
Marvin H. Eng and Firas Zahr

Mitral valve dysfunction is prevalent amongst older patients. Of those not suitable for surgical therapy, mitral transcatheter edge-to-edge repair (TEER) can treat as large proportion of patients, many are not suitable TEER candidates. As such, orthotopic transcatheter mitral valve replacement (TMVR) is an important innovation but it faces significant challenges. Orthotopic TMVR requires a prosthesis with stable anchoring, adequate sealing, minimal footprint in the left ventricle and long term durability. Multidisciplinary expertise in advanced imaging, surgery, heart failure are needed for success.

Transcatheter Mitral Valve Therapies in Patients with Mitral Annular Calcification   237
Patrick S. Kietrsunthorn, Fadi Ghrair, Aaron R. Schelegle, and Jason R. Foerst

Mitral annular calcification is a chronic process involving degeneration and calcium deposition within the fibrous skeleton of the mitral valve annulus, which can lead to mitral valve dysfunction. It can be asymptomatic, or it can have pathologic sequelae leading to cardiovascular morbidity and mortality. Mitral annular calcification is increasingly recognized with the advancement of diagnostic imaging modalities, especially in an era with a growing elderly population. Its presence poses considerable challenges in terms of surgical and transcatheter management. Multiple surgical and transcatheter techniques have been developed to overcome these challenges. New transcatheter technologies are under investigation to tackle this problem.

Transcatheter Mitral Annuloplasty: Carillon Device   249
Vinayak Nagaraja and Samir R. Kapadia

Functional mitral regurgitation (FMR) is a common valvular heart disease in the geriatric population across the United States. This patient cohort is multimorbid and often has a prohibitive risk for conventional open-heart surgery. The diverse anatomic pathology of FMR is a complex problem and unfortunately does not have a universal solution. Carillon Mitral Contour System (Cardiac Dimensions, Kirkland, WA, USA) is a new device that provides transcatheter annular remodeling. In this review article, the authors summarize the evidence for the Carillon Mitral Contour System for FMR.

Minimally Invasive Mitral Valve Repair Using Transcatheter Chordal Attachments   257
Chandan Das, Ghayth Al Awwa, Emmanuel L. Mills, and Gurion Lantz

The advent of transcatheter mitral chordal replacement techniques has offered an alternative approach that is less invasive and may be more suitable for select patients compared with surgical repair. These systems involve introducing artificial chordae, via catheter, to replace or supplement damaged or elongated natural chordae. These artificial chordae are anchored at one end to the mitral leaflet and the other end to the papillary muscle or directly to the left ventricular apex, restoring the leaflet's coaptation and reducing regurgitation. Early trials and studies suggest promising results in terms of safety and efficacy in reducing MR severity and improving symptoms.

Transcatheter Therapy for Mitral Valve Stenosis   271
Kris Kumar and Timothy Simpson

Mitral valve stenosis remains highly prevalent among the US population although with dramatically shifting demographics. The significance of rheumatic mitral disease in developing nations persists, despite improvements in preventative measures and early detection, and its presence in developed countries is still evident as observed through international migration. In addition, the substantial growth in the aging population with a heightened occurrence of concurrent cardiovascular risk factors is leading to an increased prevalence of chronic calcific degeneration and degeneration of previously repaired or replaced valves. This article aims to review various transcatheter therapies in the treatment of mitral valve stenosis.

Transcatheter Treatment of Mitral Valve Regurgitation in the Setting of   279
Concomitant Coronary or Multivalvular Heart Disease: A Focused Review
Jay Ramsay, Yicheng Tang, Jin Kyung Kim, and Antonio H. Frangieh

Treatment for mixed valve disease has historically been limited, often surgery being the only option. With the recent advancement of transcatheter therapies, percutaneous approaches are quickly becoming viable therapeutic considerations in inoperable or high-risk patients, also offering the option for a staged or same-session treatment. Guidelines are primarily focused on single-valve disease. However, patients often present with multiple pathologies. This review summarizes the data and literature on transcatheter treatment of patients with mitral regurgitation who concomitantly have aortic stenosis or regurgitation, tricuspid regurgitation, or ischemic cardiomyopathy. Pathophysiology, hemodynamics, available therapies as well as order and timing of interventions are discussed.

TRANSCATHETER MITRAL VALVES

FORTHCOMING ISSUES

July 2024
Interventions for Congenital Heart Disease
Frank F. Ing and Howaida El-Said, *Editors*

October 2024
Antiplatelet and Anticoagulation Therapy in
Cardiovascular and Pulmonary Embolism
Transcatheter Interventions
Luis Ortega Paz, *Editor*

RECENT ISSUES

January 2024
Multi-Modality Interventional Imaging
Thomas Smith, *Editor*

October 2023
Renal Disease Considerations in Coronary,
Peripheral and Structural Interventions
Shweta Bansal, *Editor*

July 2023
Pulmonary Embolism Interventions
Vikas Aggarwal, *Editor*

THE CLINICS ARE NOW AVAILABLE ONLINE!

Access your subscription at:
www.theclinics.com

PREFACE

Transcatheter Mitral Interventions: Multidisciplinary Progress at Its Best

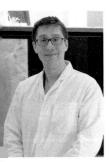
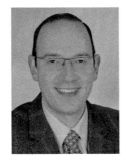

Marvin H. Eng, MD   **Firas Zahr, MD**
Editors

The widespread presence of mitral valvular pathology, particularly in elderly patients has made providing alternatives to surgical treatment a priority. Just as in transcatheter aortic valve replacement, a large unmet need is present as the prevalence of mitral pathology exceeds even that of aortic pathology. Mitral anatomy is significantly more complex than aortic valve dysfunction due its relationships with surrounding structures such as the aortic-mitral curtain, left ventricular outflow tract, coronary sinus and circumflex artery. To add confusion, mitral dysfunction can result from ventricular dysfunction despite normal leaflet morphology, therefore cardiomyopathy treatment is integrated into treating mitral disease. The diversity in leaflet pathology requires multiple tools for accurate characterization and treatment. Ultimately to comprehensively treat mitral valve disease, we require expertise in imaging, cardiomyopathy therapy, surgery and a combination of therapeutic tools.

Deeper understanding of mitral anatomy is pushing cardiac imaging to provide more detailed analysis folding in predictive treatment modeling and artificial intelligence. Each modality has had iterated significantly, mostly using sophisticated volumetric imaging tools and making 3-dimensional (3D) echocardiography and computed tomography (CT) standard of care. Lesion identification, risk assessment, therapy suitability, and implantation guidance now require dedicated imaging specialists and the integration of multiple imaging modalities.

Recognition of mitral valvular dysfunction as a symptom of ventricular disease shifts the focus of treatment to the ventricle. Therefore, the treatment armamentarium includes correct heart failure staging, optimization of medical therapy, appropriate use of resynchronization, correction of valvular regurgitation and consideration of surgically based mechanical circulatory support or transplantation. The effectiveness of halting the reciprocal positive feedback loop of ventricular failure and mitral regurgitation was illustrated in the COAPT trial making valvular therapy a cornerstone of cardiomyopathy treatment. Since the focus of treatment shifts from the valve to the ventricle, interventionalists find themselves integrating into a complex multidisciplinary team of heart failure specialists and surgeons.

Intervent Cardiol Clin 13 (2024) xiii–xiv
https://doi.org/10.1016/j.iccl.2024.01.005
2211-7458/24/© 2024 Published by Elsevier Inc.

The transcatheter therapy revolution in structural heart disease has been advancing at a dizzying pace for the last 15 years. As such, the learning curve for structural heart disease specialists has become very steep and this issue is a testament for the possible need for interventionalists to differentiate and focus similar to what is seen in cardiac surgery. In this issue, advancements in imaging, clinical management, expansion of indications, transcatheter leaflet-based repair, annuloplasty repair, and valve replacement are discussed. We are grateful for the contributions of the world class physicians in this issue and hope to provide a comprehensive layout for the current landscape of mitral interventions as well as a foundation for advancing the field.

DISCLOSURES

Marvin H. Eng is a clinical proctor for Edwards Lifesciences and Medtronic. He is on the speaker's panel for LivaNova. Firas Zahr receives research and educational grants and is a consultant for Edwards Lifesciences and Medtronic.

Marvin H. Eng, M
Division of Cardiolog
University of Arizon
Banner University Medical Cente
755 East McDowell Roa
Phoenix, AZ 85006, US

Firas Zahr, M
Division of Cardiovascular Medicin
Knight Cardiovascular Institute Cardiology Clini
Oregon Health and Science Universit
3303 South Bond Avenu
Building 1, 7th Floc
Portland, OR 97239, US

E-mail addresse:
Marvin.eng@bannerhealth.com (M.H. Eng
zahr@ohsu.edu (F. Zah

Imaging of the Mitral Valve

Pranav Chandrashekar, MD, Chandralekha Ashangari, MD,
Scott M. Chadderdon, MD*

KEYWORDS

- Mitral regurgitation • Mitral stenosis • Transthoracic echocardiography
- Transesophageal echocardiography

KEY POINTS

- Echocardiographic imaging is the foundation for the evaluation of mitral valve dysfunction.
- Transesophageal imaging is essential in providing an accurate anatomic assessment of pathology as well as more accurate quantification of valve dysfunction.
- Transesophageal imaging is required in the planning and guidance of transcatheter mitral valve repair and transcatheter mitral valve replacement procedures.
- Cardiac CT is essential in procedural planning for transcatheter mitral valve replacement procedures.
- Cardiac MRI is a useful technique for diagnosing the etiology and severity of mitral valve disease when echocardiographic data are discrepant or limited.

INTRODUCTION

Echocardiographic imaging is the foundation for evaluation of mitral valve dysfunction. The 2020 American College of Cardiology (ACC)/ American Heart Association (AHA) Guidelines for the Management of Valvular Heart Disease provides a class I recommendation for use of transthoracic echocardiography (TTE) for the baseline evaluation of mitral regurgitation (MR) and mitral stenosis to establish the diagnosis, assess for mechanism of dysfunction, and to quantify of severity of mitral valve disease.[1] Transesophageal echocardiography (TEE) plays an important role peri-procedural imaging of the mitral valve when planning either a surgical or percutaneous intervention.[2] Additionally, TEE also can provide information when there is lack of clarity in the etiology of mitral valve dysfunction and provide further insight when there may be insufficient or discordant data.

Defining the mitral anatomy is the first step of echocardiographic assessment and care should be taken to define the mitral annulus, leaflet scallops, chordae tendinae, and the papillary muscles which all contribute to the structure and the function of the mitral valve. In MR, it is important to classify the mechanism of regurgitation as either primary or secondary to help guide management. This is accomplished by evaluation of the mitral valve leaflet morphology (thickening, calcification, prolapse, or flail), mobility/motion of leaflets, mitral valve annulus size, and papillary muscle distance.[3] Primary MR is defined by degenerative/structural changes of the mitral valve leaflets and/or annulus (myxomatous, calcific, inflammatory, infectious) and most often lead to eccentric jets of MR.[4] Conversely, secondary MR results from global dilation and remodeling of the left ventricle (LV) and/or the left atrium (LA), typically resulting in central jets with normal leaflet structure. In mitral stenosis, valve anatomy assessment is critical to determine the appropriate treatment.[5] The presence of commissural fusion will help to determine if the mitral stenosis is rheumatic in etiology or degenerative due to calcification.[6] Additional anatomic information that should be obtained includes the following: leaflet thickening, leaflet calcification, mobility of leaflets, and thickening of sub-valvular apparatus as prognostic indicators of a favorable

---

Knight Cardiovascular Institute, Oregon Health & Science University, 3181 Southwest Sam Jackson Park Road, Portland, OR 97239, USA
* Corresponding author.
E-mail address: chadderd@ohsu.edu

Intervent Cardiol Clin 13 (2024) 141–153
https://doi.org/10.1016/j.iccl.2023.12.003

response to percutaneous balloon mitral valvulo-plasty of rheumatic mitral stenosis.[7] TEE imaging significantly improves spatial and temporal reso-lution for assessment of the mitral valve anatomy given the proximity of the imaging footplate to the LA and mitral annulus. This resolution also al-lows for improved 3-dimensional (3D) recon-struction which is crucial to better identify the specific anatomy and pathology of the mitral valve to aid in the selection of surgical or trans-catheter treatment options.

The utilization of Doppler echocardiography with color flow imaging, pulsed wave Doppler, and continuous wave Doppler is the gold stan-dard in the semi-quantitative and quantitative analysis of mitral valve dysfunction.[3] Doppler echocardiography allows for the determination of the speed and direction of blood flow thus enabling the echocardiographer to assess MR jet direction, vena contracta width, color flow jet area, LA to LV inflow velocities, pulmonary vein inflow patterns, and quantitatively assess effective regurgitant orifice area (EROA) by the proximal isovelocity surface area (PISA) principle.[8]

In addition to the evaluation of the mitral valve itself, echocardiography provides impor-tant adjunctive information for assessment of left ventricular size and function, right ventricular function, LA size, pulmonary artery pressures, as well as presence of concomitant valvular lesions. These findings also help to inform the hemody-namic consequences of the valve dysfunction which is used for determination of timing of intervention.[1]

Once a decision is made to proceed with intervention, the use of TEE imaging is essential as it provides a more accurate anatomic assess-ment of pathology as well as more accurate quantification of valve dysfunction.[2] For surgical intervention, TEE is the standard for imaging intraoperatively. Following mitral valve repair for MR, TEE imaging is used for detection of re-sidual MR and can lead to re-operation if resid-ual MR is greater than expected or other if complications are found. For percutaneous transcatheter interventions for MR, TEE is required for the procedure in order to guide transseptal crossing and to guide the deploy-ment of transcatheter edge-to-edge-repair (TEER) devices as well as transcatheter mitral valve replacement (TMVR) devices.

Quantification of Mitral Valve Dysfunction

Quantification of mitral valve dysfunction is important as the severity guides frequency of monitoring as well as the timing of intervention.

Echocardiography with Doppler is the most commonly used method due to the ease of use. There are several methods used to quantify the severity of MR, and a multi-parametric approach is needed to integrate the information for an accurate interpretation (Table 1). It is pru-dent to be aware of the limitations of these indi-vidual methods and these can affect accuracy. Loading conditions can also alter the severity if significantly different between studies if the blood pressure varies significantly. Particularly in secondary MR there can be a large variation in severity depending on the afterload and intra-vascular fluid status of the patient. We will re-view the methods of quantification of mitral valve dysfunction using echocardiography.

Mitral Regurgitation
Color flow Doppler imaging

The use of the color flow Doppler jet is the first indicator of whether a patient has MR based on the direction and timing of the color jet.[9] The jet area or the ratio of the jet area/LA area measured from the apical views is the simplest method for visualization of severity; however, there are numerous technical, anatomic, and physiologic factors that limit its accuracy. The Nyquist limit setting can significantly alter the size of the jet (Fig. 1). Additionally, an eccentric jet may appear smaller in area due to its approx-imation on the left atrial chamber wall. However, a central jet with area greater than 50% of the LA suggests severe MR.

The vena contracta is the narrowest portion of a jet that is present just downstream from the orifice (Fig. 2A) and its cross-sectional area rep-resents a measure of the eEROA. Severity of MR is quantified based on the width of the vena con-tracta (VCW). It should be measured in the para-sternal long axis view zoomed in on mitral valve and the convergence zone needs to be visual-ized. VCW is used in a semi-quantitative fashion where a VCW with measurements greater than 0.7 cm usually correlating with a regurgitant vol-ume greater than 60 mL and EROA greater than 0.4 cm². VCW can be measured for eccentric jets as well.

Flow convergence or PISA method is based on the principle of the creation of hemispheric shells of increasing velocity as blood approaches a regurgitant orifice (Fig. 2B–D). This allows for estimation of the EROA and regurgitant volume and is the preferred method for central regurgi-tation. Accuracy in the PISA method requires optimization of acquisition by aligning the direc-tion of regurgitant flow with the ultrasound beam in order to be as co-axial as possible to

Table 1
Echocardiographic features that indicate severe mitral regurgitation

	Severe Mitral Regurgitation Parameters	Limitations
Quantitative assessment		
Effective regurgitant orifice area	≥ 0.4 cm2	Eccentric or multiple jets limit accuracy
Regurgitant volume	≥ 60 mL	
Regurgitant fraction	≥50%	
Semi quantitative		
Pulmonary vein inflow Doppler profile	Systolic flow reversal	Eccentric jet may be directed at a single pulmonary vein
2D vena contracta width	≥ 0.7 cm	Multiple jets limit use
3D vena contracta area	> 0.4 cm2	Prone to blooming artifact
Mitral inflow Doppler profile	E-wave dominant ≥ 1.2 m/sec	Dependent on left ventricle and left atrium compliance
Color flow jet area	≥ 50% of left atrium	Eccentric jet area may not appear to be large
Supporting features		
Left ventricle size and function	Dilated left ventricle. LV ejection fraction <50%	
Left atrial volume	Severely dilated (LA volume index>55 mL/m2)	
Mitral regurgitation Doppler pattern	Dense triangular pattern	
Abnormal valve anatomy	Large flail leaflet Large perforation of leaflet	

create a full 180° hemispheric arc.[10] If an MR jet is eccentric, the subvalvular PISA hemisphere may be constrained which leads to a larger PISA radius, though multiplying by angle correction factor (α/180) can account for this.[11] When multiple MR jets are present, individual PISA measurement should be made for each jet to summate the total EROA.

Continuous wave and pulsed wave Doppler
The use of continuous wave (CW) and pulsed wave (PW) Doppler methods can give indirect clues to the severity of MR.

- Qualitative assessment of the density of the CW Doppler of the MR jet can reflect the proportion of red blood cells that are reflecting the signal. Additionally, a more triangular contour can suggest hemodynamic significance, but these are not sensitive parameters.
- PW Doppler recordings of the mitral inflow velocity at the level of the leaflet tips aligned coaxially with the ultrasound beam will demonstrate an E wave and an A-wave if there is atrial contraction. An E velocity greater than 1.2 m/sec is a supportive sign of severe MR. However, the E-wave velocity also depends on filling pressures and compliance of the LV so this must be considered when analyzing this Doppler profile. This also can be variable in setting of irregular cycles such as with atrial fibrillation.
- PW Doppler of the pulmonary vein inflow pattern can sometimes be difficult to accurately obtain with TTE imaging; however, the presence of systolic flow reversal in more than one is specific for severe MR.[3] Eccentric jets that are not severe but directed into a pulmonary vein can falsely suggest severe MR.

The integration of 2D measurements with PW Doppler recordings of flow velocity can be used to derive stroke volume across a single valve. LV

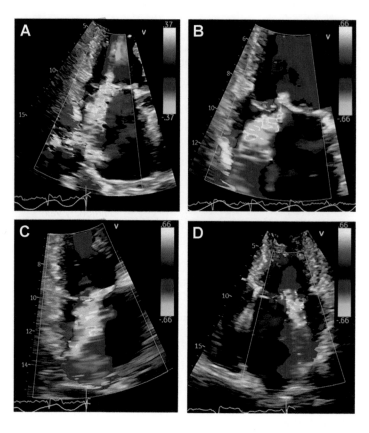

Fig. 1. 2D Transthoracic Echo Color Doppler Imaging of Mitral Valve Regurgitation. (*A*) Apical 3 chamber view showing large eccentric posterior directed jet of Mitral Regurgitation (MR) overestimated in severity as Nyquist Limit at 37 cm/s. (*B*) Apical 3 chamber zoomed view at Nyquist limit of 66 cm/s with moderate to severe MR (*C*) Apical 2 chamber view of MR jet less than 50% of left atrium (*D*) Apical 4 chamber view of MR jet less than 50% of left atrium.

forward stroke volume is derived from measurement of the LV outflow tract diameter from 2D imaging to estimate the cross-sectional area (assuming it is circular) and PW Doppler of the LV outflow tract. Stroke volume across the mitral valve is derived by measuring the MV annulus on 2D imaging and PW Doppler at the level of the MV annulus. The regurgitant volume can be derived by subtracting the LV forward stroke volume through a competent aortic valve from the stroke volume across the mitral valve (Fig. 3). Mitral annular area can be calculated through use of 3D multi-planar reconstruction (MPR) of the annulus with direct planimetry. However, if this technique is not readily available, a single 2D measurement of the annulus diameter in the commissure-to-commissure view on TEE has a 97% accuracy with 3D MPR.[12] Stroke volume across the mitral valve can also be estimated by measurement of LV volumes, subtracting the end-systolic LV volume from the end-diastolic LV volume. The use of echo contrast can improve accuracy of LV volume measurement, though, this method requires meticulous 2D measurements as small errors will be magnified due to squaring of diameters when calculating cross sectional area. Additionally, the presence of aortic regurgitation makes this method invalid; however, forward stroke volume across the pulmonic valve can be used as a surrogate if this can be accurately measured.[3]

Mitral Stenosis

The assessment of severity of mitral stenosis is graded based on estimation of the mitral valve area (MVA) by both direct and indirect methods as well as estimation of hemodynamic impact using the transmitral pressure gradients and measuring pulmonary artery pressures. Anatomic features of the MV anatomy and presence of concomitant MR also play a role. The etiology of mitral stenosis will impact assessment of severity due to the pathophysiological differences in development of the stenosis in rheumatic disease compared to mitral annular calcification. Severe MS is now considered to be less than 1.5 cm2 according to the updated 2020 ACC/AHA guidelines for valvular heart disease.[1]

Mitral valve area estimation

- MVA by planimetry: The direct measurement of MVA by planimetry is completed by tracing of the elliptical MV orifice in parasternal short axis view that is

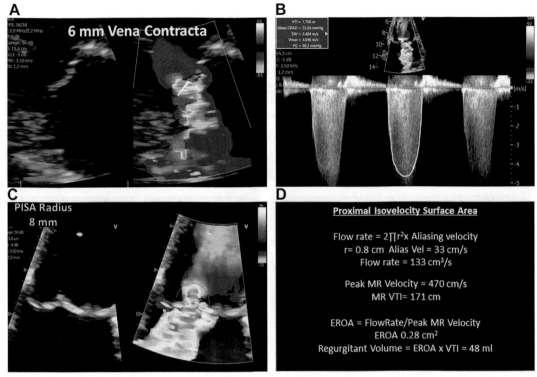

Fig. 2. 2D Transthoracic Echo Color Doppler Imaging of Mitral Valve Vena Contracta, PISA Radius and Equation. (A) 2D TTE color Doppler compare image of parasternal long axis view zoomed on mitral valve that demonstrates 6 mm vena contracta. (B) 2D TTE 4 chamber color compared zoomed image of mitral valve with Nyquist Limit shifted to 33 cm/s for EROA quantification by PISA analysis. (C) Continuous wave Doppler of peak regurgitant jet velocity across the mitral valve. (D) PISA calculation. EROA, effective regurgitant orifice area; PISA, proximal surface isovelocity area.

obtained from the orthogonal image of the biplane cursor across the mitral valve leaflet tips in mid-diastole (Fig. 4A). This measurement correlates well with the anatomic mitral valve area and is not dependent on assumptions related to flow conditions or chamber compliance.[13] While this 2D planimetry TTE method has been validated in rheumatic MS, it is more difficult degenerative MS due to distortion of orifice geometry and calcification. Conversely, 3D MPR from TTE or TEE can be utilized for more precise alignment of the short axis plan at the leaflet tips provided an appropriate frame rate and adequate visualization (Fig. 4B).

- MVA by PISA method: There is convergence of diastolic mitral flow on the atrial side of the mitral valve that allows for the measurement of mitral flow and calculation of MVA based the utilization of the PISA method.[14] For MS assessment, the color baseline is shifted toward the LV (direction of mitral inflow)

and the mitral flow rate is calculated as: $(2\pi r^2$ x Nyquist shifted aliasing velocity) divided by peak mitral inflow velocity by CW Doppler (Fig. 4C, D). It should be noted there are often concerns for accuracy in measuring the radius of the convergent flow as well as the need for angle correction of the flow relative to the opening angle of the mitral leaflet.[14]

- MVA by continuity equation: This method relies on estimation of LV forward stroke volume using PW Doppler which should equal the volume of diastolic mitral flow. Inherent limitations are the errors in measurement and being unable to be applied in cases with atrial fibrillation or significant aortic insufficiency and concomitant moderate or more MR.
- MVA by pressure half time: This method should be applied to those with rheumatic MS and is less reliable in those with degenerative MS or those with abnormal left atrial compliance or LV diastolic function.[15] The relation of

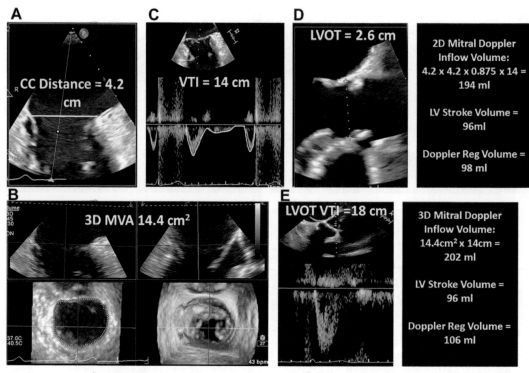

Fig. 3. 2D and 3D MPR TEE Imaging of Mitral Valve Annulus for Calculation of Regurgitant Volume. (*A*) Commissure-to-Commissure (CC) distance of mitral annulus where area is assumed to be circular and calculates to 13.8 cm², (*B*) 3D multi-planar reconstruction (MPR) direct planimetry of the mitral valve annulus measures 14.4 cm² (4% difference from CC method), (*C*) Pulse wave Doppler at mitral valve annulus with velocity time integral (VTI) of 14 cm, (*D*) Left ventricular outflow track (LVOT) measurement acquired as biplane image from the center of the aortic valve at 60°/150° (*E*) Transgastric off axis Left ventricular outflow track (LVOT) velocity time integral (VTI) for calculation of left ventricular stroke volume. Mitral valve inflow volume minus left ventricular stroke volume = mitral regurgitant volume. Regurgitant volume divided by the mitral regurgitation peak regurgitation velocity = Effective Regurgitant Orifice Area (EROA) though calculation not shown in figure.

pressure half time relies on the slow decline of transmitral velocity reflecting the valvular impedance to passive flow.[16] In degenerative MS there is a rapid fall in velocity and often comorbidities affecting chamber compliance making this unreliable.

Transmitral gradients

The mean transmitral gradient is reliably assessed by CW Doppler but is not the best marker of severity of MS since it is dependent on the transmitral flow rate which is influenced by the heart rate, cardiac output, and associated MR.[14] Thus, this should be used in conjunction with other variables of severity and taken into account with abnormal LV compliance. At heart rates from 60 to 80 bpm, a mean transmitral gradient greater than 10 mm Hg is suggestive of severe MS.

Role of Exercise Echocardiography

The use of exercise to complement echocardiographic imaging allows for the unmasking of symptoms due to valve dysfunction and helps to establish a true functional capacity. There are technical limitations related to obtaining accurate images at peak exercise. The use of the supine bicycle allows for improved imaging quality. For MR exercise echocardiography can assess the ability to augment LV function in primary MR, increases in EROA in secondary MR, and increase in pulmonary artery pressures in asymptomatic severe primary MR all of which can provide clinically relevant prognostic information.[17] In mitral stenosis there can be often discordant measurements of severity with atypical symptoms. Exercise testing can help to discern the hemodynamic impact of mitral stenosis with exertion. Limitations of exercise testing are that thresholds for severity at peak exercise are not well defined and are based on low quality evidence.

Role of Transesophageal Imaging for Mitral Valve Dysfunction

As detailed earlier, there are several limitations to the accurate noninvasive assessment of the

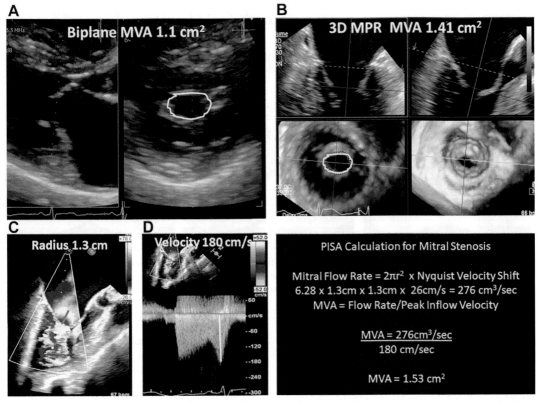

Fig. 4. 2D and 3D MPR TEE Imaging of Mitral Valve for Quantification of Mitral Stenosis in a Patient with Rheumatic Mitral Stenosis. (A) Biplane across the parasternal long axis view at mitral leaflet tips in mid-diastole with planimetry measurement in orthogonal short plane axis. (B) 3D multi-planar reconstruction (MPR) of mitral valve leaflet tips in mid-diastole with increased specificity of mitral valve area. (C) Mitral inflow velocity proximal surface isovelocity area (PISA) radius measurement. (D) Mitral inflow peak velocity by continuous wave (CW) Doppler and resultant PISA calculated MVA.

severity of MR and MS. Eccentric flow can underestimate the severity of MR by color Doppler as well as for estimation of PISA radius. Similarly, due to mitral annular calcification, there can be difficulty in identifying the anatomy of the mitral valve tips to determine the MVA by planimetry. These issues can often be improved due to the superior spatial and temporal resolution of transesophageal echocardiographic imaging. Additionally, TEE provides additional information that is not possible to be accurately obtained by transthoracic imaging and is required for planning and guidance of transseptal procedures as well as transcatheter mitral valve repair strategies that are commercially available and transcatheter mitral valve replacement options that are available in clinical trials.

Anatomic assessment of the mitral valve apparatus

Defining the anatomy of the mitral valve is important for determination of etiology and the mechanism of mitral valve dysfunction and

TEE imaging provides superior resolution. Spatial resolution in echocardiography improves with the areas of interest being imaged being at a right angle to the beam, hence the TEE probe should be manipulated such that the mitral annulus is as perpendicular to the ultrasound beam as possible. The mid-esophageal commissural view at 50 to 70° is a key view for mitral valve imaging (Fig. 5). The P3-A2-P1 scallops are viewed and using biplane imaging at each scallop allows for visualization of A3-P3, A2-P2, and A1-P1 scallops individually. In order to obtain an ideal mid-esophageal commissural view, there should be symmetric display of the papillary muscle heads and chords. Additional views at 0 to 20°, 80 to 100°, 120 to 140°, and 150 to 170° can be used to image the coaptation of individual scallops, particularly with MR to help view eccentric regurgitation jets. Transgastric view allows for visualization of the short axis orientation of the mitral valve or for assessment of subvalvular apparatus when there is shadowing from significant mitral annular calcification.

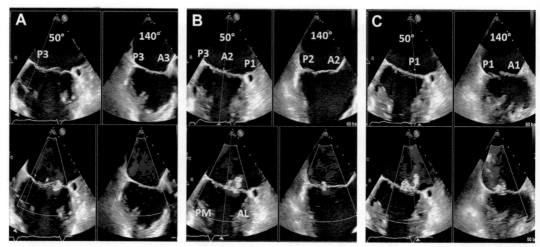

Fig. 5. 2D Transesophageal echocardiography (TEE) with Biplane Sweep of Mitral Valve with and without Color. (*A*) Biplane imaging in the mitral valve commissural view with and without color at 50° across P3 with P3/A3 scallops displayed on orthogonal angle at 140°. (*B*) Biplane imaging of A2 at 50° with corresponding orthogonal view of P2/A2 scallops. (*C*) Biplane imaging of P1 at 50° with corresponding orthogonal view of P1/A1 scallops. A, anterior; AL, anterior-lateral; P, posterior; PM, posterior-medial.

An additional advantage of TEE imaging is the ability to capture high resolution 3-dimensional images of the mitral valve apparatus.[18] A 3-dimensional image allows for the entire valve to be visualized in a single view to identify the location and extent of abnormal scallops as well as allowing simultaneous examination of both leaflets and visualization of adjacent anatomic structures (Fig. 6A). Color Doppler can be added to the 3D image for identification of blood flow (Fig. 6B). Acquisition of high resolution 3-dimensional imaging should start with obtaining a high quality 2-dimensional image from the mid-esophageal commissural view. If the patient is in sinus rhythm without ectopy additional temporal resolution can be achieved with multi-beat acquisition (although if there is respiratory motion this can result in a stich artifact). Post processing can be performed on a 3-dimensional volume set with multi-planar reconstruction.

Assessment of mitral valve dysfunction using transesophageal imaging

TEE imaging helps to provide additional information for the severity of mitral valve dysfunction and is most useful when there is discordant or

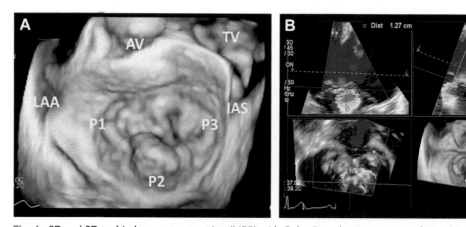

Fig. 6. 3D and 3D multi-planar reconstruction (MPR) with Color Doppler Assessment of Mitral Regurgitation. (*A*) 3D En-face view of the mitral valve in surgeons view with aorta at top of image demonstrates myxomatous mitral valve disease with bi-leaflet prolapse and severe prolapse of P2 segment. (*B*) 3D En-face view with color Doppler flow and MPR with 3D PISA (proximal surface isovelocity area) quantification of the severity mitral regurgitation. AV, aortic valve; IAS, intra-atrial septum; LAA, Left atrial appendage; TV, tricuspid valve.

insufficient information obtained with transthoracic imaging. For mitral stenosis using multiplanar reconstruction of a 3D image, the mitral valve area estimation by planimetry is superior to transthoracic imaging from the short axis view as the tips of the leaflets can be more accurately identified.[19] This can be particularly helpful in the presence of calcification in degenerative MS where traditional indirect measurements of severity have not been validated compared to rheumatic MS.[16]

For MR, in addition to accurate identification of leaflet pathology, the assessment of severity of MR utilizes color Doppler imaging as described earlier and shown earlier (see Figs. 2 and 6). TEE imaging improves accuracy when the regurgitant jet is eccentric to allow for aligning of the beam in the direction of the jet or when there are multiple jets. The use of multiplanar reconstruction of a 3D volume set with addition of color Doppler allows for a more accurate estimation of the vena contracta area as well as regurgitant orifice area through alignment in the direction of the eccentric jet or through multiple jets if present. Another key advantage of TEE imaging is the ability to view the pulmonary veins for interrogation of the color Doppler profile for assessment of systolic flow reversal. The bifurcation of left upper and left lower pulmonary veins can be viewed from the mid-esophageal 120-degree view by rotating the probe leftward from the mitral valve and is typically adjacent to the left atrial appendage. From this view rotating the probe rightward past the superior vena cava in the superior vena cava/inferior vena cava view typically allows for the identification of the right upper pulmonary vein. Advancing the probe and reducing the multiplane angle around 40 to 80° can allow for the identification of the right

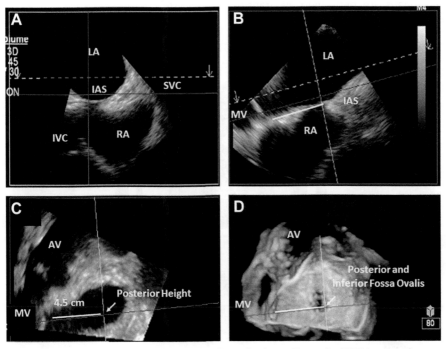

Fig. 7. 3D multi-planar reconstruction (MPR) Transesophageal echocardiography (TEE) imaging for assessment of the inter-atrial septum (IAS) and guidance of mitral valve TEER procedure. (A) 3D MPR evaluation of the IAS to measure distance from transseptal puncture site to the mitral annulus. The left upper green plane images the superior vena cava/ inferir vena cava (SVC/IVC) view red orthogonal plane placed at the inferior border of the fossa ovalis and the blue short axis is aligned parallel to the IAS. (B) The right upper red plan images the 4 chamber view of the heart across the IAS with visualization of the base of the mitral valve (MV). The of the posterior height of a transseptal puncture can then be performed on the red plane, noted at 4.5 cm, and can be adjusted with 3D evaluation of the IAS from an LA vantage point as demonstrated in box C and box D. (C) The blue plane short axis image of the IAS has been Z-rotated 90° counterclockwise to the SVC is at the top aspect of the screen and the IVC is at the bottom aspect of the screen. This places the MV annulus to the left part of the screen to appreciate potential different trajectories if the transseptal puncture is more superior or inferior in the IAS. (D) 3D rendering of the IAS and fossa ovalis from left atrial view for 3D visualization of relationship of the fossa to the mitral annulus for transcatheter mitral procedure planning.

lower pulmonary vein although lower angles may be required.

Use of transesophageal imaging for transcatheter mitral valve interventions

TEER of the mitral valve for severe MR has a class 2A recommendation in the correct clinical setting.[1] For TEER, the identification of leaflet length, coaptation gap, and flail gap is needed to determine if a TEER device may be deployed reliably. Novel methods for transcatheter mitral valve replacement are currently being studied in clinical trials for treatment of MR as well as degenerative mitral stenosis.[20,21] TEE imaging is essential for both assessment of feasibility as well as intraprocedural guidance.[1] Multi-planar reconstruction is used for assessment of the mitral valve area for TEER treatment and can also be utilized to measure the mitral annular area and perimeter for transcatheter valve replacement options in clinical trials. As mitral valve interventions are performed via transfemoral venous route, appropriate site and safe transseptal access to the LA is essential. From the mid-esophageal bi-caval view at 110° the interatrial septum is visualized with the addition of biplane and 3D. Optimal site is decided based on distance in the superior/inferior axis to prevent injury to the aortic root as well in the anterior/posterior axis to ensure there is enough height from the mitral valve annulus to allow for maneuverability of the transcatheter system for accurate deployment (Fig. 7). Once transseptal access has been obtained, TEE provides guidance for the correct positioning, trajectory, and alignment of transcatheter repair and replacement devices (Fig. 8). It also provides real-time feedback on any hemodynamic concern that could develop during the procedure from development of pericardial effusion or impact of the transcatheter delivery systems on the mitral valve leaflets or chordae that can contribute to significant MR, hypotension and tachycardia.

Computed tomography for analysis of mitral valve dysfunction

Cardiac Multi-Detector Computed Tomography (MDCT) plays a significant role in the assessment of the mitral valve and is complementary to

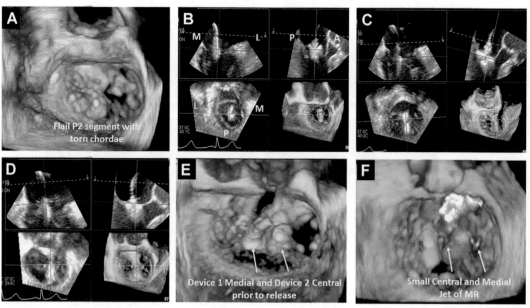

Fig. 8. 3D Transesophageal echocardiography (TEE) multi-planar reconstruction (MPR) and 3D Doppler Color use in Mitral Transcatheter-Edge-to-Edge- Repair (TEER) Procedure. (A) 3D imaging of En-face view of mitral valve with fail P2 with torn chordae from anterior lateral papillary muscle. (B) 3D MPR assessment for device positioning (medial section of flail), trajectory to leaflets in the medial (M) to lateral (L) (green plane) and anterior (A) to posterior (P) (red plane) with Z-rotation of aorta to 12 o'clock position and short axis blue line on TEER device for appropriate device alignment along coaptation plane (blue plane and 3D image). (C) 3D MPR imaging of leaflet engagement on TEER device, (D) closure of TEER device with A/P leaflet insertion on red plane and tissue-bridge demonstrated on 3D view, (E) 3D En-face view of medical device 1 and placement of second TEER device just lateral to close flail segment, (F) 3D color Doppler En-face view demonstrating small residual central and medial jet of mitral regurgitation that in total is mild in severity.

echocardiography prior to transcatheter intervention. MDCT is performed by electrocardiographic gating with a retrospective acquisition during the entire cardiac cycle. It is then reconstructed in multiple cardiac phases throughout the cardiac cycle. The reconstruction is performed in 5% increments with corresponding RR interval and using the smallest slice thickness possible thus facilitating excellent spatial resolution in multiple cardiac phases throughout systole and diastole for differential measurements.[22] Cardiac MDCT is useful to assess the mitral annular dimensions and mitral annular calcification, length of the leaflets, papillary muscle distance, LV outflow tract (LVOT) area. CT also plays a major role in defining the landing zone for TMV procedures. It provides detailed information on the extent and severity of annular calcium, which can help determine device suitability as well. For the mitral valve annulus, 3D measurement of the annulus area, perimeter, and septal-lateral and inter-commissural distance should be performed for appropriate valve selection and sizing. Accurate measurement of the annulus is important for appropriate sizing of the TMVR device as inaccurate sizing can lead to device embolization and

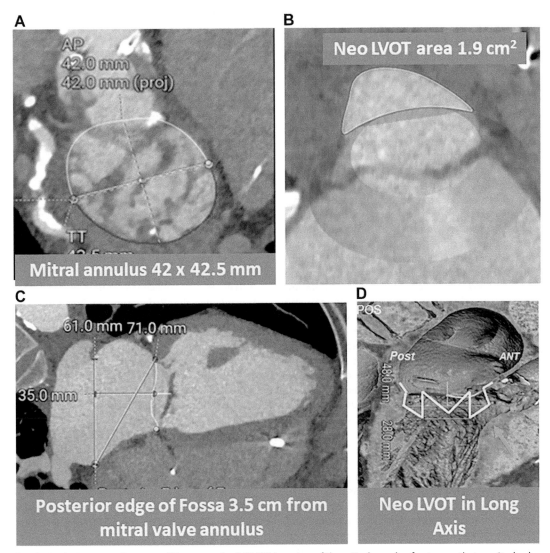

Fig. 9. Multi-Detector Computed Tomography (MDCT) imaging of the mitral annulus for transcatheter mitral valve replacement (TMVR) procedural planning. (A) Mitral annular diameters in systole for valve sizing. (B) Neo-left ventricle outflow tract (LVOT) measurement of 1.9 cm² with virtual valve in mitral annulus, (C) 4 chamber analysis of left arterium (LA) sizing (6 cm wide) and intra-atrial septum for height posterior to mitral valve annulus (3.5 cm) as well as diagonal length to lateral mitral annulus (7 cm), (D) 3D long axis rendering of virtual valve in mitral annulus and representative LVOT view.

annular rupture by undersizing and oversizing respectively. While the specificity of 3D MDCT is preferred for mitral procedural planning, 3D TEE sizing of the mitral annulus in the context of TMVR has shown good intra-observer and inter-observer reproducibility and a high correlation with MDCT sizing of the mitral annulus.[23] Fig. 9 demonstrates MDCT sizing of the mitral annulus, left ventricular outflow tract, and LA and inter-atrial septum measurements prior to TMVR.

Magnetic resonance imaging of the mitral valve

While echocardiography is the first line imaging test for the assessment of MR, cardiac MRI is complimentary, noninvasive imaging modality that provides a comprehensive assessment of the mitral valve. Cardiac MRI provides accurate flow quantification of MR, provides precise volumetric assessments, and also provides assessment of myocardial scar or fibrosis that is important diagnostically and prognostically. Cardiac MR also helps to assess the anatomy of the mitral valve in primary MR and anatomy and the function of the LV in secondary MR.[24–26] Cardiac MR can also accurately measure the severity of the MR by various methods; (1) phase contrast sequences of aortic flow and calculating the mitral regurgitant volume, (2) direct quantification of MR through the use of a trans-annular phase contrast sequence acquisition, and (3) via stroke volume differences in the LV and the RV.[27,28] Thus, when echocardiographic data are limited or discrepant, cardiac MR can be exceedingly useful in the diagnosis and management of patients with mitral valve dysfunction. Limiting factors in the use of cardiac MR include the length of examination as well as artifacts and imaging safety concerns where there are cardiac implanted devices such as pacemakers, defibrillators, and previous implanted surgical valves or transcatheter devices.

SUMMARY

Echocardiography is the foundation for the assessment of valvular heart disease as it provides detailed qualitative and quantitative analysis of chambers sizes and morphology and etiology of valvular dysfunction. There is no significant risk with transthoracic imaging whereas the adjunctive imaging modalities of CT and MR can be contra-indicated in patients with significant renal dysfunction, but the each clearly have their role in procedural planning and precise volume and regurgitation quantification,

respectively. The ubiquity, reliability, and speed of diagnostic imaging with echocardiography will keep it at the forefront of cardiac valvular assessment as it continues to evolve and progress in technology yearly. TEE is, at this point, the indispensable imaging modality in transcatheter mitral procedures, though advancements in intra-cardiac echocardiographic imaging are progressing and will undoubtedly have applications in the future for patients unable to tolerate TEE procedures. Regardless of the imaging modality chosen, it is imperative to understand the underlying pathology, morphology, and etiology of mitral valvular dysfunction for appropriate diagnosis and treatment strategies for patients.

DISCLOSURE

S.M. Chadderdon is a consultant for Edwards Lifesciences and Medtronic Inc. Dr S.M. Chadderdon receives imaging grant support from GE Healthcare, United Kingdom, Siemens Healthineers, Germany, and Phillips. Dr P. Chandrashekar and Dr C. Ashangari have no disclosures.

REFERENCES

1. Otto CM, Nishimura, Bonow, et al. 2020 ACC/AHA Guideline for the Management of Patients With Valvular Heart Disease: Executive Summary: A Report of the American College of Cardiology/American Heart Association Joint Committee on Clinical Practice Guidelines. Circulation 2021;143(5):e35–71.
2. Hahn RT, Saric, Faletra, et al. Recommended Standards for the Performance of Transesophageal Echocardiographic Screening for Structural Heart Intervention: From the American Society of Echocardiography. J Am Soc Echocardiogr 2022;35(1):1–76.
3. Zoghbi WA, Adams, Bonow, et al. Recommendations for Noninvasive Evaluation of Native Valvular Regurgitation: A Report from the American Society of Echocardiography Developed in Collaboration with the Society for Cardiovascular Magnetic Resonance. J Am Soc Echocardiogr 2017;30(4):303–71.
4. Stone GW, Vahanian, Adams, et al. Clinical Trial Design Principles and Endpoint Definitions for Transcatheter Mitral Valve Repair and Replacement: Part 1: Clinical Trial Design Principles: A Consensus Document From the Mitral Valve Academic Research Consortium. J Am Coll Cardiol 2015;66(3):278–307.
5. Baumgartner H, Hung, Bermejo, et al. Echocardiographic assessment of valve stenosis: EAE/ASE recommendations for clinical practice. J Am Soc Echocardiogr 2009;22(1):1–2 [quiz: 101–2].
6. Veasy LG. Time to take soundings in acute rheumatic fever. Lancet 2001;357(9273):1994–5.

7. Wilkins GT, Weyman, Abascal, et al. Percutaneous balloon dilatation of the mitral valve: an analysis of echocardiographic variables related to outcome and the mechanism of dilatation. Br Heart J 1988; 60(4):299–308.

8. Vandervoort PM, Rivera, Mele, et al. Application of color Doppler flow mapping to calculate effective regurgitant orifice area. An in vitro study and initial clinical observations. Circulation 1993;88(3):1150–6.

9. Zoghbi WA, Enriquez-Sarano, Foster, et al. Recommendations for evaluation of the severity of native valvular regurgitation with two-dimensional and Doppler echocardiography. J Am Soc Echocardiogr 2003;16(7):777–802.

10. Grayburn PA, Weissman NJ, Zamorano JL. Quantitation of Mitral Regurgitation. Circulation 2012; 126(16):2005–17.

11. Pu M, Vandervoort, Griffin, et al. Quantification of mitral regurgitation by the proximal convergence method using transesophageal echocardiography. Clinical validation of a geometric correction for proximal flow constraint. Circulation 1995;92(8): 2169–77.

12. Hyodo E, Iwata, Tugcu, et al. Accurate measurement of mitral annular area by using single and biplane linear measurements: comparison of conventional methods with the three-dimensional planimetric method. Eur Heart J Cardiovasc Imaging 2011;13(7):605–11.

13. Faletra F, Pezzano, Fusco, et al. Measurement of mitral valve area in mitral stenosis: four echocardiographic methods compared with direct measurement of anatomic orifices. J Am Coll Cardiol 1996;28(5):1190–7.

14. Rahimtoola SH, Durairaj, Mehra, et al. Current evaluation and management of patients with mitral stenosis. Circulation 2002;106(10):1183–8.

15. Gonzalez MA, Child JS, Krivokapich J. Comparison of two-dimensional and Doppler echocardiography and intracardiac hemodynamics for quantification of mitral stenosis. Am J Cardiol 1987;60(4):327–32.

16. Reddy YNV, Murgo JP, Nishimura RA. Complexity of Defining Severe "Stenosis" From Mitral Annular Calcification. Circulation 2019;140(7):523–5.

17. Leung DY, Griffin, Stewart, et al. Left ventricular function after valve repair for chronic mitral regurgitation: predictive value of preoperative assessment of contractile reserve by exercise echocardiography. J Am Coll Cardiol 1996;28(5):1198–205.

18. Tsang W, Lang RM. Three-dimensional Echocardiography Is Essential for Intraoperative Assessment of Mitral Regurgitation. Circulation 2013;128(6): 643–52.

19. Zamorano J, Cordeiro, Sugeng, et al. Real-time three-dimensional echocardiography for rheumatic mitral valve stenosis evaluation: an accurate and novel approach. J Am Coll Cardiol 2004;43(11): 2091–6.

20. Eleid MF, Wang, Pursnani, et al. 2-Year Outcomes of Transcatheter Mitral Valve Replacement in Patients With Annular Calcification, Rings, and Bioprostheses. J Am Coll Cardiol 2022;80(23):2171–83.

21. Zahr F, Song HK, Chadderdon S, et al. 1-Year Outcomes Following Transfemoral Transseptal Transcatheter Mitral Valve Replacement: Intrepid TMVR Early Feasibility Study Results. JACC Cardiovasc Interv 2023;16(23):2868–79.

22. Blanke P, Dvir, Cheung, et al. A simplified D-shaped model of the mitral annulus to facilitate CT-based sizing before transcatheter mitral valve implantation. J Cardiovasc Comput Tomogr 2014; 8(6):459–67.

23. Mak GJ, Blanke, Ong, et al. Three-Dimensional Echocardiography Compared With Computed Tomography to Determine Mitral Annulus Size Before Transcatheter Mitral Valve Implantation. Circ Cardiovasc Imaging 2016;9(6):e004176.

24. Han Y, Peters, Salton, et al. Cardiovascular magnetic resonance characterization of mitral valve prolapse. JACC Cardiovasc Imaging 2008;1(3): 294–303.

25. Perazzolo Marra M, Basso, De Lazzari, et al. Morphofunctional Abnormalities of Mitral Annulus and Arrhythmic Mitral Valve Prolapse. Circ Cardiovasc Imaging 2016;9(8):e005030.

26. Sturla F, Onorati, Puppini, et al. Dynamic and quantitative evaluation of degenerative mitral valve disease: a dedicated framework based on cardiac magnetic resonance imaging. J Thorac Dis 2017; 9(Suppl 4):S225–38.

27. Mehta NK, Kim, Siden, et al. Utility of cardiac magnetic resonance for evaluation of mitral regurgitation prior to mitral valve surgery. J Thorac Dis 2017;9(Suppl 4):S246–56.

28. Uretsky S, Gillam, Lang, et al. Discordance between echocardiography and MRI in the assessment of mitral regurgitation severity: a prospective multicenter trial. J Am Coll Cardiol 2015;65(11):1078–88.

Mitral Transcatheter Edge-to-Edge Repair
Advancing Treatment Options for Degenerative Mitral Regurgitation

Salman Zahid, MD[a], Jasmine Anjali Garg, MD[b],
Ahmed Altibi, MD[a], Harsh Golwala, MD[a],*

KEYWORDS

- Mitral valve repair • TEER • Mitral valve regurgitation • Degenerative MR
- Transcatheter edge-to-edge repair

KEY POINTS

- Mitral transcatheter edge to edge repair (M-TEER) is a recommended treatment of choice for severe symptomatic degenerative mitral regurgitation (MR) in patients with prohibitive surgical risk.
- The ideal M-TEER anatomy encompasses central (A2/P2) MR, intact leaflets without clefts or perforations, absence of calcification in the grasping area, mitral valve area (MVA) greater than 4.0 cm^2, posterior leaflet length greater than 10 mm, normal leaflet mobility and thickness, flail width less than 15 mm, and a flail gap of no more than 10 mm.
- The emergence of next-generation M-TEER devices may extend its utility to more challenging cases in comprehensive heart valve centers, encompassing conditions like Barlow disease, commissural leaks (A1/P1, A3/P3), wide flail, MVA less than 4.0 cm^2, moderate-severe mitral annular calcification, and calcification in the leaflet capture zone.

INTRODUCTION

Over the past decade, degenerative mitral regurgitation (DMR) has gained extensive interest because of innovative technologies emerging in the treatment of the same.[1] MR is prevalent, affecting around 10% of those over the age of 75, with a 2% to 3% incidence in the United States.[2–4] Untreated MR leads to adverse heart remodeling, resulting in left ventricular dysfunction, pulmonary hypertension, and heart failure (HF) syndrome, negatively affecting quality of life and mortality.[1,3,5,6] Despite surgical valve repair/replacement treatment being the standard of care, many severe MR patients face unmet clinical needs because of high or prohibitive surgical risks, often related to age and frailty.[7] This has led to the emergence of transcatheter therapies for high- and prohibitive-risk surgical patients, most notably mitral transcatheter edge-to-edge repair (M-TEER) devices.

In the historic timeline of surgical treatment, Alfieri's technique in 1991 initiated the approximation of the middle scallops of anterior and posterior leaflets' creating a bifurcated orifice mitral valve.[8] Subsequently, St. Goar and colleagues in 2003 introduced an endovascular approach, detailing the successful restoration

---

Funding: None.
[a] Department of Cardiovascular Medicine, Knight Cardiovascular Institute, Oregon Health and Science University, 3161 SW Pavillon Loop, Portland, OR 97239, USA; [b] Department of Medicine, Westchester Medical Center, 100 Woods Road, Valhalla, NY 10595, USA
* Corresponding author. Interventional Cardiology, Knight Cardiovascular Institute, Oregon Health & Science University, 3161 SW Pavillon Loop, UHN62, Portland, OR 97239, USA
E-mail address: golwala@ohsu.edu

Intervent Cardiol Clin 13 (2024) 155–165
https://doi.org/10.1016/j.iccl.2024.01.001
2211-7458/24/© 2024 Elsevier Inc. All rights reserved.

of leaflet coaptation using a clip.[9] The MitraClip (Abbott Vascular, Minnesota, MN)), a breakthrough technology in clinical practice, gained prominence with the case of Octalina Mendoza from Caracas, Venezuela.[10] The device subsequently received US Food and Drug Administration (FDA) approval for DMR in 2013 following promising results in the EVEREST (Endovascular Valve Edge-to-Edge REpair Study) trials.[11] More recently, PASCAL Transcatheter Valve Repair System (Edwards LifeSciences, Irvine, California) obtained a CE mark approval in Europe and was FDA-approved in 2022.[12,13]

This article addresses key aspects of M-TEER for DMR, such as clinical trial evidence, patient evaluation and selection, procedural strategies, and an in-depth understanding of commercially available M-TEER devices.

PATIENT EVALUATION

After conducting a thorough assessment of the patient's history, symptoms, and physical examination, the initial step for evaluating DMR involves a comprehensive transthoracic echocardiogram (TTE). TTE employs qualitative, quantitative, and semiquantitative criteria using 2-dimensional, 3-dimensional, and Doppler assessments, as outlined in Table 1 to assess the etiology and severity of MR. When dealing with DMR, it is crucial to consider hemodynamic factors that can impact the assessment of MR severity. For example, in conditions like myxomatous degeneration of the mitral valve (MV) prolapse, when systemic blood pressure is elevated, the evaluation of MR severity must account for hemodynamic conditions and blood flow velocities across the valve. This is vital because even if the effective regurgitant orifice area remains consistent, the actual volume of regurgitation can vary. High systemic blood pressure might lead to an overestimation of MR.[14,15] In contrast, the eccentricity of the MR jet, known as the Coanda effect, can potentially result in the underestimation of the severity of MR during TTE assessment.

Most patients with severe MR should undergo a thorough transesophageal echocardiogram (TEE) assessment to understand the mechanism of MR and assess the feasibility of the M-TEER procedure, especially the anatomy of interatrial septum for trans-septal access. The bi-commissural view (60–70° midesophageal view) provides an overview of the valve layout from medial to lateral, while the biplane long-axis views (120–150° midesophageal views) define the anatomy of the anterior and posterior leaflets. 3-dimensional TEE is particularly useful in conditions like prolapse and flail segments, allowing for evaluation from the surgeon's view. The ventricular view helps understand the subchordal support mechanism, obtain proximal isovelocity surface area (PISA) measurements, and assess for clefts or indentations in the leaflets. 3-dimensional MV planimetry is valuable in cases with mixed valvular disease. More recently, 3-dimensional multiplanar reconstruction has been extremely useful and enhances the ability to simultaneously view multiple imaging planes (see Fig. 2A–C). In select cases, performing a dedicated gated cardiac computed tomography (CT) scan aids in understanding the MV apparatus by delineating the degree and extent of MV calcification. Finally, in cases where TEE is challenging or contraindicated, MRI can provide an accurate volumetric assessment of MR severity.

PATIENT SELECTION

An essential step in selecting patients for M-TEER involves defining the individual patient's anatomy of the MV apparatus using high-quality TEE. This apparatus comprises the MV leaflets (anterior and posterior), the mitral annulus, and the subchordal apparatus, including the papillary muscles and the chordae tendinea (Fig. 1).

The initial focus in DMR treatment through M-TEER is a thorough assessment of leaflets.[16] The posterior leaflet adopts a crescent shape, encompassing roughly two-thirds of the annular circumference. In contrast, the broader anterior leaflet covers the remaining one-third and maintains an anatomic relationship with the left and noncoronary aortic cusp anteriorly. The posterior leaflet is further divided into 3 well defined scallops: P1 (lateral), P2 (central), and P3 (medial), while the anterior leaflet has less well defined 3 scallops: A1 (lateral), A2 (central), and A3 (medial) (Fig. 1; Fig. 2A–C). An important consideration for M-TEER is determining the length of the posterior leaflet, which significantly influences device selection and procedural intricacies. Ideally, a posterior leaflet length exceeding 10 mm is optimal; lengths between 6 and 10 mm are suboptimal, and lengths below 6 mm present technical challenges in M-TEER. Additionally, the presence of clefts or indentations within the posterior leaflet, particularly if they extend beyond half of the leaflet's height, requires attention, as these clefts or indentations can lead to residual MR after addressing the primary A2/P2 pathology.[16,17] Finally, assessing the degree of calcification within both leaflets, especially in the region where grasping for TEER occurs, is essential. An uncalcified

Table 1
Assessment of mitral valve regurgitation severity

Qualitative Assessment	Criteria for Severe MR	TTE Images
Jet area	Jet area more than 50% of the LA area	
Continuous flow doppler	Dense holosystolic and triangular jet	
Hemispheric flow convergence	Large holosystolic flow convergence	
Semi-quantitative assessment		
Mitral inflow pattern	E-wave dominant (a predominant A wave will exclude severe MR) E wave velocity >1.2 m/s	
Pulmonary vein flow	Systolic flow reversal	
Vena contracta (VC) width	VC more than 0.7 cm	

(continued on next page)

Qualitative Assessment	Criteria for Severe MR	TTE Images
Table 1 *(continued)*		
Qualitative Assessment	**Criteria for Severe MR**	**TTE Images**
Quantitative assessment		Equation for calculation
Regurgitant fraction	>50%	Regurgitant fraction = (Regurgitant Volume/Forward Stroke Volume) * 100
Effective regurgitant orifice area (cm^2)	>0.40 cm2	EROA = $2\pi r^2$ * Vmax/Vm
Regurgitant volume (mL)	60 mL	RV = EROA * VTI (VTI is the velocity time integral of the regurgitant jet)

Abbreviations: EROA, effective regurgitant orifice area; LA, left atrium; MR, Mitral regurgitation; PISA, proximal isovelocity surface area; r, Radius of the hemisphere at the origin of the regurgitant jet; RV, regurgitant volume; TEE, transesophageal echocardiography; VC, venacontracta; Vm, Alias velocity (Nyquist limit) of the color Doppler used; Vmax, Peak velocity of the regurgitant jet; VTI, velocity time integral.

grasping zone is ideal, as calcifications within this area reduce the procedure's success rate. Fig. 3 summarizes the optimal and suboptimal MV anatomy for M-TEER.[15–17]

The mitral annulus, primarily composed of fibrous tissue, acts as a barrier separating the left ventricle (LV) and the left atrium (LA). It is crucial to evaluate the presence of calcification within the annular region, as extensive calcifications not only decrease the MV area but also hinder the annulus from returning to its natural shape after TEER, negatively affecting the TEER results.[14,15,17]

MV apparatus usually involves 2 papillary muscles that include the posteromedial papillary muscles, attached to the medial segment of the MV leaflets, and the anterolateral papillary muscle affixed to the lateral counterpart of the leaflets

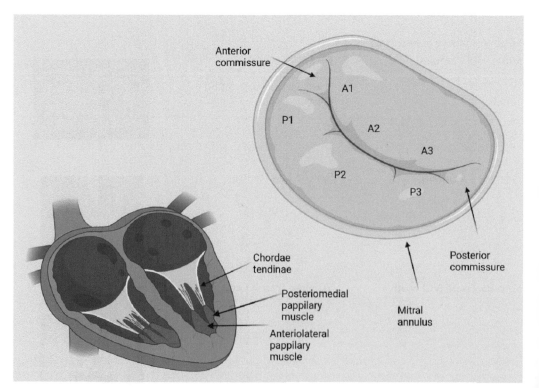

Fig. 1. MV apparatus. A1, A2, and A3 refer to scallops of the anterior mitral leaflet. P1, P2, and P3 A3 refer to scallops of the posterior mitral leaflet.

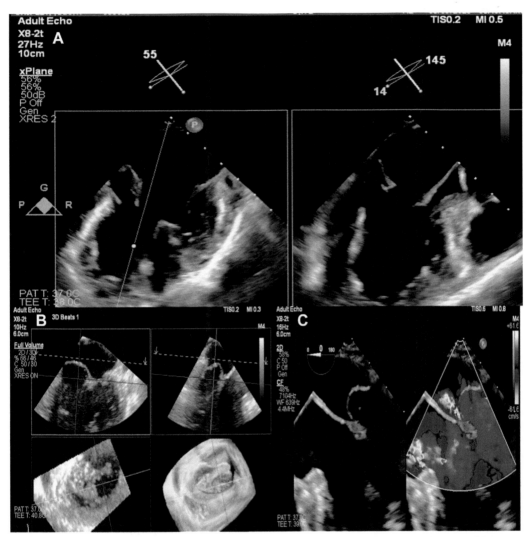

Fig. 2. M-TEER assessment using echocardiography. (A) The commissural view on the left side and midesophageal long axis view on the right side shows the MV apparatus including the anterior MV leaflet, posterior MV leaflet, anterolateral papillary muscle, and the posteromedial papillary muscle. (B) 3-dimensional ECHO shows prolapse of the posterior mitral leaflet. (C) Color compare mode shows predominant prolapse of the P2-A2 with central MR jet.

(see Figs. 1 and 2A–C). It is important to note that chordae tendineae from both anterolateral and posteromedial papillary muscles extend to both leaflets, increasing the risk of entrapment during TEER procedures. The density of the chordal apparatus is highest at the medial and lateral commissures; therefore significant caution should be taken when treating these regions. Sufficient chordal support significantly enhances the chances of a successful M-TEER outcome, while inadequate chordal support, as seen in cases such as papillary muscle dysfunction following a myocardial infarction, can make the M-TEER procedure challenging[14,17]

COMMERCIALLY APPROVED DEVICES

MitraClip Device

The MitraClip system comprises 2 key components: a steerable guide catheter (SGC) and a clip delivery system (CDS) with a detachable clip. The SGC boasts a tapered design, starting at 25 French at its proximal end and narrowing to 23 French at the distal end. The distal end of the SGC is curved, and it features a single knob with positive and negative adjustments, allowing for additional curving or straightening of the catheter's tip as needed. The guide handle can be rotated in either a clockwise or counterclockwise direction, enabling posterior

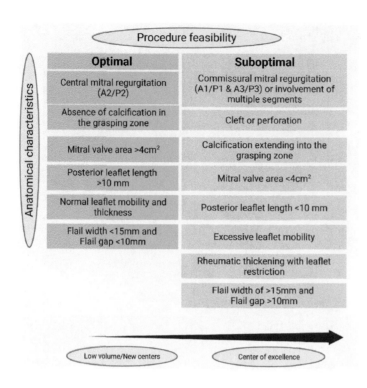

Fig. 3. Optimal and Suboptimal anatomy for M-TEER.

or anterior movement for precise guide positioning. Turning the knob in the positive direction adds more curvature to the SGC's tip, which is particularly useful for correcting an aorta hugger position, while turning it in the negative direction straightens the tip and helps loose height in certain circumstances. This combination enables precise manipulation of the clip in multiple planes, enhancing the effectiveness of M-TEER (Fig. 4A, B).[14,18]

The CDS is inserted into the SGC, which is then advanced into the left atrium. The CDS is equipped with controls for precise device positioning, including the M/L knob for medial-or lateral trajectory and the A/P knob for antero-posterior movement (see Fig. 4A, B).

The fourth-generation MitraClip, known as MitraClip G4, brings significant enhancements with controlled gripper actuation. This technology allows for simultaneous or independent grasping of leaflets, ensuring improved leaflet insertion. Furthermore, the MitraClip G4 devices provide 4 different clip sizes, offering tailored M-TEER options to accommodate various MV apparatus anatomies. Currently available devices include NT, XT, NTW, and XTW (see Fig. 4A, B). These devices are constructed using a cobalt-chromium metal alloy and consist of 2 rigid arms that incorporate flexible nitinol grippers. These grippers are equipped with either 4 hooks (NT/NTW) or 6 hooks (XT/XTW) arranged longitudinally. The increased arm length of the XT/XTW versions allows for addressing more extensive coaptation gaps and leaflet flails, surpassing the stringent criteria for inclusion in the EVEREST study.

PASCAL SYSTEM

The more recently approved PASCAL system comprises of 3 essential components, including a guide sheath, a steerable sheath, and an implant catheter that harbors the CLASPs (Fig. 5).[16,19]

The importance of paddles lies in their role in achieving leaflet approximation, while clasps allow for independent leaflet capture, enabling precise leaflet insertion adjustment. Notably, the PASCAL implant distinguishes itself from the MitraClip system by utilizing a single row of grippers in each clasp, a deviation from the typical 4 to 6 rows in the MitraClip system. In addition, the central spacer serves to reduce tension, effectively occupying the regurgitant orifice, thus minimizing MR. Another advantage of the PASCAL implant is its elongation capability, ensuring safe retraction from the subvalvular apparatus and reducing the risk of chordal damage.

The PASCAL implant, available in 2 sizes (PASCAL: 10 mm width and PASCAL Ace:

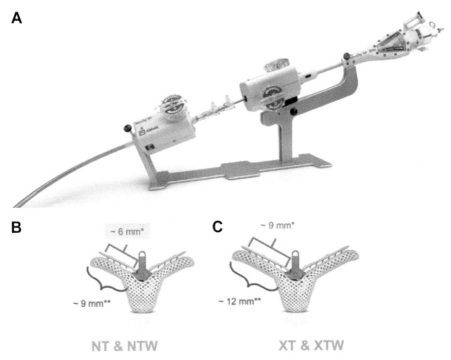

Fig. 4. MitraClip devices. (A) Mitraclip system, (B) NT and NTW clip; (C) XT and XTW clip. Abbott, Abbott 'A', and MitraClip are trademarks of Abbott or its related companies. Reproduced with permission of Abbott, © 2023. All rights reserved.

6 mm width), encompasses 2 paddles, 2 clasps, and a central spacer (see Fig. 5).

CLINICAL TRIAL EVIDENCE FOR MITRAL TRANSCATHETER EDGE-TO-EDGE REPAIR

The EVEREST II study, a pivotal investigation focusing on M-TEER versus conventional surgery in patients with degenerative MR, described an array of MV anatomic characteristics linked to improved outcomes and mitigation of severe DMR.[7,20,21] Although M-TEER showed lower efficacy in reducing the severity of mitral MR compared with surgery, it was linked to a superior safety profile and comparable clinical outcomes. The EXPAND registry conducted an analysis of real-world patient outcomes involving individuals with significant MR who underwent treatment

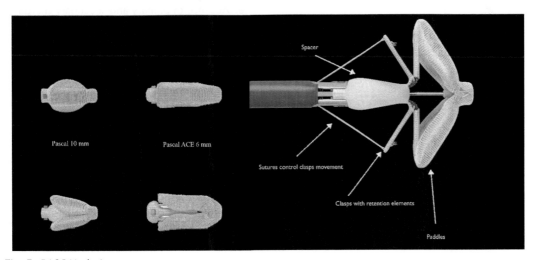

Fig. 5. PASCAL device system.

Table 2
Major inclusion and exclusion criteria for mitral transcatheter edge to edge repair based on the EVEREST trial

Major Inclusion Criteria	Major Exclusion Criteria
The primary regurgitant flow stems from the malcoaptation of the A2 and P2 scallops of the MV If a secondary regurgitant jet is present, it should be deemed clinically inconsequential.	Myocardial infarction occurring in the 12 weeks leading up to the planned treatment
Symptomatic MR with >25% left ventricular ejection fraction (LVEF) and left ventricular end-systolic diameter (LVESD) ≤55 mm	Clinical indication for additional cardiac surgical procedures
If MR is asymptomatic then 1 or more of the following: a. LVEF 25% to 60% b. LVESD ≥40 mm c. New onset of atrial fibrillation d. Pulmonary hypertension (defined as pulmonary artery systolic pressure >50 mm Hg at rest or >60 mm Hg with exercise)	Any endovascular, therapeutic, interventional, or surgical procedure conducted in the 30 days preceding
The operator assesses the feasibility of trans-septal catheterization and is deemed feasible	LVEF <25%, and/or LVESD >55 mm
Eligible for surgery involving mitral valve repair or replacement, including the use of cardiopulmonary bypass	MV orifice area <4.0 cm^2
	If leaflet tethering is present, coaptation depth >11 mm, or vertical coaptation length is < 2 mm If leaflet flail is present, the width of the flail segment is > 15 mm and flail gap is > 10 mm
	Leaflet anatomy that precludes clip implantation or proper clip positioning to sufficiently reduce MR may include: a. Calcification in the grasping zone of the A2 and/or P2 scallops b. Cleft of A2 or P2 scallops c. More than 1 anatomic criteria are dimensionally near the exclusion limits d. Bileaflet flail or severe bileaflet prolapse e. Absence of primary and secondary chordal support f. Previous mitral valve surgery or valvuloplasty, or the presence of a currently implanted mechanical prosthetic valve or ventricular assist device; echocardiographic evidence of intracardiac mass, thrombus, or vegetation g. History of atrial septal defect or patent foramen ovale associated with clinical symptoms h. History of or currently active rheumatic heart disease or endocarditis

Feldman T, Foster E, Glower DD, Kar S, Rinaldi MJ, Fail PS, Smalling RW, Siegel R, Rose GA, Engeron E, Loghin C, Trento A, Skipper ER, Fudge T, Letsou GV, Massaro JM, Mauri L; EVEREST II Investigators. Percutaneous repair or surgery for mitral regurgitation. N Engl J Med. 2011 Apr 14;364(15):1395-406. https://doi.org/10.1056/NEJMoa1009355. Epub 2011 Apr 4. Erratum in: N Engl J Med. 2011 Jul 14;365(2):189. Glower, Donald G [corrected to Glower, Donald D]. PMID: 21463154.

with the next-generation MitraClip NTR and XTR systems (included wider clip sizes of NTW and XTW).[22] At 30 days follow-up, there was a substantial reduction in MR compared with baseline, with 98% of patients achieving MR levels of 2+ or lower, and 91% achieving MR levels of 1+ or lower. Notably, there were significant enhancements in functional capacity and quality of life, as 83% of patients attained New York Heart Association (NYHA) functional class I or II. These findings from the real world registry affirmed MR reduction outcomes and provided strong evidence of the safety and efficacy of these devices. Based on findings of the EVEREST II(21) landmark trial, the 2020 valvular heart disease guidelines by the American Heart Association and the American College of Cardiology gave M-TEER a Class IIa recommendation for treatment of DMR in patients at high or prohibitive surgical risk, provided their MV anatomy is favorable.[15,23] Similarly, the 2021 guidelines emanating from the European Society of Cardiology endorsed a Class IIb classification, designated for patients with either inoperable circumstances or elevated surgical risk.[16,24] These recommendations, however, hinge upon the absence of substantial anatomic constraints as outlined in the exclusion criteria of the EVEREST trial (Table 2).

The CLASP IID trial (NCT03706833) studied the safety and efficacy of the Edwards PASCAL Transcatheter Valve Repair System compared with the MitraClip system in individuals with severe symptomatic DMR at prohibitive surgical risk.[25] One hundred eighty individuals with severe DMR (3+ or 4+) were randomly allocated, with two-thirds receiving the PASCAL system and one-third undergoing treatment with the Mitra-Clip. In this device comparison trial, the PASCAL system demonstrated noninferiority compared with the MitraClip system for the primary endpoints of major adverse event rate and achieving MR severity ≤2+ in terms of safety and effectiveness. Additionally, the study revealed significant improvements in functional status and quality of life for patients in both treatment groups. Notably, the proportion of individuals with MR of no more than 1+ in the PASCAL group retained durable repair from the time of discharge to the 6-month follow-up (87.2% at discharge and 83.7% at 6 months; $P = 0.317$).[25]

SUITABLE VERSUS UNSUITABLE ANATOMY FOR MITRAL TRANSCATHETER EDGE-TO-EDGE REPAIR

The success of M-TEER is significantly influenced by the favorable anatomy of the MV. The EVEREST criteria, as outlined in Table 2, establish the guidelines for determining eligibility based on MV anatomy.[21]

Although the initial[21] criteria were stringent in their inclusion and exclusion, the introduction of the newer-generation MitraClip G4, featuring wider and longer clip arms (NTW, XTW) as shown in Fig. 4A, B, and the availability of various sizes of the PASCAL devices have expanded the scope of treatable cases (see Fig. 5). These advancements now enable the successful treatment of more complex anatomic issues, such as larger flail gaps and commissural gaps, particularly in experienced centers (see Fig. 3).

To aid in assessing the suitability of M-TEER, a color-coded system has been proposed to classify anatomy as optimal or suboptimal.[26] (see Fig. 3). Although these guidelines are valuable in predicting the success of mitral TEER therapy, it is essential to acknowledge that outcomes are also influenced by the learning curve, individual experience, and the expertise of the valve center, particularly in cases falling within the yellow zone.

TRANSESOPHAGEAL ECHOCARDIOGRAM VERSUS INTRACARDIAC ECHOCARDIOGRAPHY-GUIDED TRANSCATHETER EDGE TO EDGE REPAIR, EMERGING IMAGING MODALITIES

TEE currently serves as the standard method for imaging M-TEER. Nevertheless, individuals who are at high risk for general anesthesia or those whose conditions make TEE unsuitable have limited treatment alternatives. Conditions that might contraindicate the use of TEE encompass sizable hiatal hernias, cervical spine disorders, and esophageal ailments such as strictures, and Barrett esophagus.[27] In scenarios where TEE is not feasible, 4-dimensional intracardiac echocardiography (ICE) presents itself as a viable technology.[28] By utilizing 4-dimensional ICE, clinicians can acquire real-time volumetric images and employ multiplanar reconstruction to guide the M-TEER procedure during the intervention.[29]

It is established that ICE and TEE each carry inherent drawbacks. For instance, TEE is associated with a higher incidence of esophageal injuries and complications related to gastrointestinal bleeding, while ICE may be linked to an increased occurrence of vascular complications because of the requirement for extra access.[30,31] Comprehensive investigations are warranted in this domain to systematically examine and compare the safety and feasibility aspects of both modalities.

SUMMARY

In conclusion, M-TEER stands as the preferred treatment for severe symptomatic degenerative MR in patients facing prohibitive surgical risk. For optimal M-TEER outcomes, the ideal anatomic criteria include central MR (A2/P2), intact leaflets without clefts or perforations, an absence of calcification in the grasping area, a MVA greater than 4 cm^2, posterior leaflet length exceeding 10 mm, normal leaflet mobility and thickness, flail width less than 15 mm, and a flail gap not exceeding 10 mm. Furthermore, the evolving landscape of next-generation M-TEER devices may expand its applicability to more complex cases, such as Barlow disease, commissural leaks (A1/P1, A3/P3), wide flail, MVA less than 4 cm^2, moderate-severe mitral annular calcification, and calcification in the leaflet capture zone. This underscores the potential for broader utilization in comprehensive heart valve centers.

CLINICS CARE POINTS

- M-TEER offers a viable option for moderate-to-severe degenerative MR treatment in patients with prohibitive surgical risk.
- Precise MV anatomy and mechanism assessment are pivotal for procedural success.
- Advanced M-TEER devices address anatomically challenging degenerative MR cases.
- ICE-guided TEER is an alternative imaging approach that demands substantial operator expertise.

DISCLOSURES

None. H. Golwala serves as an advisory consultant for Medtronic and Boston Scientific.

REFERENCES

1. Del Forno B, De Bonis M, Agricola E, et al. Mitral valve regurgitation: a disease with a wide spectrum of therapeutic options. Nat Rev Cardiol 2020; 17(12):807–27.
2. Nkomo VT, Gardin JM, Skelton TN, et al. Burden of valvular heart diseases: a population-based study. Lancet 2006;368(9540):1005–11.
3. Foster E. Mitral regurgitation due to degenerative mitral-valve disease. N Engl J Med 2010;363(2): 156–65.
4. Freed LA, Levy D, Levine RA, et al. Prevalence and clinical outcome of mitral-valve prolapse. N Engl J Med 1999;341(1):1–7.
5. Dziadzko V, Clavel MA, Dziadzko M, et al. Outcome and undertreatment of mitral regurgitation: a community cohort study. Lancet 2018 Mar;391(10124): 960–9.
6. Abdallah ES, Yogesh NVR, Rick AN. Mitral valve regurgitation in the contemporary era. JACC Cardiovasc Imaging 2018;11(4):628–43.
7. Feldman T, Kar S, Rinaldi M, et al. Percutaneous mitral repair with the MitraClip system: safety and midterm durability in the initial EVEREST (Endovascular Valve Edge-to-Edge REpair Study) cohort. J Am Coll Cardiol 2009;54(8):686–94.
8. Alfieri O, Maisano F, De Bonis M, et al. The Double-orifice technique in mitral valve repair: a simple solution for complex problems. J Thorac Cardiovasc Surg 2001;122(4):674–81.
9. St Goar FG, Fann JI, Komtebedde J, et al. Endovascular edge-to-edge mitral valve repair: short-term results in a porcine model. Circulation 2003; 108(16):1990–3.
10. Abbott. The MitraClip Story. 2016. Available at: https://www.abbott.com/corpnewsroom/products-and-innovation/the-mitraclip-story.html. [Accessed 21 July 2023].
11. US food & Drug Administration. Premarket Approval (PMA) MitraClip delivery system. 2013. Available at: https://www.accessdata.fda.gov/scripts/cdrh/cfdocs/cfpma/pma.cfm?id=P100009. [Accessed 21 July 2023].
12. Webb JG, Hensey M, Szerlip M, et al. 1-year outcomes for transcatheter repair in patients with mitral regurgitation from the CLASP study. JACC Cardiovasc Interv 2020;13(20):2344–57.
13. TCTMD, FDA Approves PASCAL TEER device for degenerative MR, Available at: https://www.tctmd.com/news/fda-approves-pascal-teer-device-degenerative-mr, Accessed October 23, 2023. 2022.
14. Reza Reyaldeen RM. Basic evaluation of mitral regurgitaiton. In: Asgar AW, Rogers JH, editors. Transcatheter edge-to-edge repair. Washington, DC: The Society of Cardiovascular Angiography and Interventions; 2022.
15. Burkhand G, Mackensen EGS. Patient selection for transcatheter mitral leaflet repair. In: Asgar AW, Rogers JH, editors. Transcatheter edge-to-edge repair. Washington, DC: The Society of Cardiovascular Angiography and Interventions; 2022.
16. Jörg H.J.S.T., Marianna A., Nicole K.J.S.M. and Fabien P., Mitral valve transcatheter edge-to-edge repair, EuroIntervention, 18 (12), 2023, 957–976 . Available at: https://eurointervention.pcronline.com/article/mitral-valve-transcatheter-edge-to-edge-repair. Accessed October 23, 2023.

17. Layoun H, Harb SC, Krishnaswamy A, et al. Patient selection for mitral transcatheter edge-to-edge repair. Methodist Debakey Cardiovasc J 2023;19(3):26–36.

18. Trevor Simard MG. A user's guide to the MitraClip device. In: Asgar AW, Rogers JH, editors. Transcatheter edge-to-edge repair. Washington, DC: The Society of Coronary Angiography and Interventions; 2022.

19. Whisenant B, Zahr F. The PASCAL transcatheter valve repair system: a user's guide. Structural Heart 2023;7(5).

20. Glower D, Ailawadi G, Argenziano M, et al. EVEREST II randomized clinical trial: predictors of mitral valve replacement in de novo surgery or after the MitraClip procedure. J Thorac Cardiovasc Surg 2012;143(4 Suppl):S60–3.

21. Feldman T, Foster E, Glower DD, et al. Percutaneous repair or surgery for mitral regurgitation. N Engl J Med 2011;364(15):1395–406.

22. Stephan von BR HRJ, Paul M, PM J, et al. Real-world outcomes of fourth-generation mitral transcatheter repair. JACC Cardiovasc Interv 2023. https://doi.org/10.1016/j.jcin.2023.05.013.

23. Otto CM, Nishimura RA, Bonow RO, et al. 2020 ACC/AHA guideline for the management of patients with valvular heart disease: executive summary: a report of the American College of Cardiology/American Heart Association Joint Committee on Clinical Practice Guidelines. Circulation 2021;143(5). e35–71.

24. Vahanian A, Beyersdorf F, Praz F, et al. 2021 ESC/EACTS guidelines for the management of valvular heart disease: developed by the Task Force for the Management of Valvular Heart Disease of the European Society of Cardiology (ESC) and the European Association for Cardio-Thoracic Surgery (EACTS). Eur Heart J 2022. https://doi.org/10.1093/eurheartj/ehab395.

25. Lim DS, Smith RL, Gillam LD, et al. Randomized comparison of transcatheter edge-to-edge repair for degenerative mitral regurgitation in prohibitive surgical risk patients. JACC Cardiovasc Interv 2022;15(24):2523–36.

26. Lim D, Herrmann H, Grayburn P, et al. Consensus document on non-suitability for transcatheter mitral valve repair by edge-to-edge therapy. Structural Heart 2021;227–33.

27. Hilberath JN, Oakes DA, Shernan SK, et al. Safety of transesophageal echocardiography. J Am Soc Echocardiogr 2010;23(11):1111–5.

28. BD I, Kyle L, Patita S, et al. 3D intracardiac echocardiography in mitral transcatheter edge-to-edge repair. JACC Case Rep 2022;4(13):780–6.

29. Pham TH, Tso J, Sanchez CE, et al. Volumetric intracardiac echocardiogram-guided mitraclip in patients intolerant to transesophageal echocardiogram: results from a multicenter registry. J Soc Cardiovasc Angiography Interv 2023;2(3):100594.

30. Freitas-Ferraz AB, Rodés-Cabau J, Junquera Vega L, et al. Transesophageal echocardiography complications associated with interventional cardiology procedures. Am Heart J 2020;221:19–28.

31. Zahid S, Gowda S, Hashem A, et al. Feasibility and safety of intracardiac echocardiography use in transcatheter left atrial appendage closure procedures. J Society for Cardiovascular Angiography & Interventions 2022;1(6):100510.

Functional Mitral Regurgitation
Patient Selection and Optimization

Pooja Prasad, MD[a], Pranav Chandrashekar, MD[b],
Harsh Golwala, MD[b], Conrad J. Macon, MD[b],
Johannes Steiner, MD[b],*

KEYWORDS

- Functional mitral regurgitation • Secondary mitral regurgitation • Heart failure
- Transcatheter edge-to-edge repair

KEY POINTS

- Functional mitral regurgitation (FMR) commonly occurs with all heart failure (HF) syndromes independent of their left ventricular ejection fraction, can accelerate maladaptive remodeling, and portends a poor prognosis.
- FMR can favorably respond to conventional pharmacologic and device-based HF therapies.
- Percutaneous transcatheter edge-to-edge repair using commercially approved devices can be performed successfully and with favorable long-term outcomes in carefully selected FMR patients, who are nonresponders to conventional HF therapies.
- A multidisciplinary complex valve team assessment is key for triaging FMR patients toward the optimal device-based, therapeutic options.

INTRODUCTION: BURDEN AND PROGNOSIS ACROSS SPECTRUM OF HEART FAILURE

Functional mitral regurgitation (FMR) occurs commonly among all subgroups of heart failure (HF) independent of ejection fraction. The prevalence of severe FMR is most substantial among patients with heart failure with reduced ejection fraction (HFrEF) affecting nearly a third of patients.[1] In a large observational cohort study of 13,223 patients with FMR, severe regurgitation was most common among patients with HFrEF but was associated with increased mortality regardless of the HF type (midrange, preserved and reduced ejection fraction). Moderate FMR or greater is independently associated with reduced survival and recurrent hospitalization, indicating that FMR should not be considered just a mere consequence of left ventricular (LV) dysfunction but a significant predictor of survival. Furthermore, severe FMR was rarely intervened on with low rates of surgical valve repair (7%) or replacement (5%) and even transcatheter repair (4%), clearly demonstrating an opportunity for the expansion of transcatheter repair in this aging population with multiple comorbidities and increased procedural risk.[2]

In this review, we discuss the unique pathophysiologic mechanisms of FMR, the medical management and ultimately patient selection for currently available transcatheter mitral valve (MV) repair systems from a HF perspective.

DIFFERENT MECHANISMS AND PATHOPHYSIOLOGIC CONSEQUENCES

The MV is a 3-dimensional-shaped structure with a saddle-shape morphology that optimizes leaflet curvature and minimizes leaflet stress, balancing

a Division of Cardiology, University of California-San Francisco, 505 Parnassus Avenue, Suite M1182, Box 0124, San Francisco, CA 94143, USA; b Knight Cardiovascular Institute, Oregon Health & Science University, 3161 SW Pavilion Loop, Portland, OR 97239, USA
* Corresponding author.
E-mail address: steinejo@ohsu.edu

Intervent Cardiol Clin 13 (2024) 167–182
https://doi.org/10.1016/j.iccl.2023.11.001
2211-7458/24/© 2023 Elsevier Inc. All rights reserved.

2 counteracting forces: displacement of the MV leaflets toward the left atrium and the tethering forces from the chordae tendinae pulling the leaflets toward the LV during systole.[3] An imbalance in the tethering and closing forces can result in incomplete coaptation of the MV leaflets and varying degrees of FMR.[4] Eventually, FMR transitions from a marker of HF to actually contributing to the disease process and volume-overloaded state.[5] We can subdivide FMR in 3 distinct phenotypes, although an overlap frequently occurs.

Ventricular-Functional Mitral Regurgitation
The most frequent form of FMR, ventricular-functional mitral regurgitation (MR) occurs due to LV remodeling from ischemic or nonischemic cardiomyopathy that prevents leaflet coaptation.[5] Global ventricular and in particular mitral annulus dilation alter the position and dynamics of the papillary muscles,[4] which can cause symmetric tethering of the MV leaflets and ultimately the characteristic, elliptical, central mitral regurgitation (Carpentier type I). This subset of patients is thought to be the more likely to respond to medical therapy and cardiac resynchronization therapy (CRT).[6]

Ischemic Mitral Regurgitation
In contrast, ischemic MR refers to posteriorly directed MR from posterior leaflet tethering (Carpentier type IIIb), which classically occurs in the setting of inferior wall motion abnormalities from myocardial infarction.[6] The presence of isolated posterior leaflet tethering presents an opportunity for targeted surgical intervention. The prevalence of ischemic MR ranges from 11% to 59% of patients after a myocardial infarction.[7]

Atrial Functional Mitral Regurgitation
In the absence of ventricular dysfunction and enlargement, left atrial enlargement with subsequent mitral annular dilatation and straightening can cause functional MR due to the loss of concavity from tethered MV leaflets.[5] The most common clinical scenarios for atrial functional MR (AFMR) are HF with preserved ejection fraction (HFpEF) and chronic atrial fibrillation (AF).[8] However, AFMR also likely contributes to the MR in patients with ventricular-functional MR who have concurrent atrial remodeling.[6]

DIAGNOSIS OF FUNCTIONAL MITRAL REGURGITATION
Echocardiographic Criteria and Common Pitfalls
As a widely accessible and noninvasive tool, transthoracic echocardiogram (TTE) remains the primary modality for FMR diagnosis with transesophogeal echocardiogram (TEE) used when TTE quality is inconclusive or for planning and guiding invasive procedures. Of note, relying on TEE under general anesthesia has been shown to underestimate the severity of FMR likely due to lower blood pressures and altered loading conditions in this dynamic lesion.[9,10] Per the American Society of Echocardiography (ASE) guidelines, identifying the mechanism of MR is highlighted as a priority in echocardiographic evaluation. Apart from semiquantitative metrics in the form of vena contracta, mitral inflow velocity, regurgitant jet size in relation to the left atrium, pulmonary vein systolic flow reversal or blunting, and LV remodeling, quantitative assessments are frequently necessary. An estimated effective orifice area (EROA) greater than 0.3 cm^2 or a regurgitant volume (RVol) of greater than 45 mL would be consistent with at least moderate-severe mitral regurgitation especially if coupled with an elliptical orifice.[4,11]

There are multiple special considerations in the diagnosis of FMR. The velocity of the MR jet is often lower due to a low-flow state, the EROA is frequently elliptical or crescent shaped rather than hemispheric, and compared with primary MR, a lower EROA of greater than 0.2 cm^2 is associated with worse outcomes.[12] However, of note the definition for severe secondary MR remains the same as for primary MR (ERO $\geq 0.4 \text{ cm}^2$ and RVol ≥ 60 mL) according to ASE guidelines.[13] Finally, chamber size, mitral E and A velocities, and pulmonary artery pressures are often related to the underlying disease process rather than functional MR, thus, limiting the weight of these factors in diagnosis.[12] Therefore, European guidelines adjusted the definition of severe FMR by lowering EROA and RVol cutoffs from 0.4 to 0.2 cm^2 and from 60 to 30 mL, respectively, also highlighting the intrinsic limitations and lack of precision of 2-dimensional echo structural and Doppler parameters.[14]

Exercise-Induced Mitral Regurgitation
Dynamic FMR can be observed in around 25% of patients. Although exercise-induced severe MR has been associated with worse exercise capacity and acute pulmonary edema, it remains underdiagnosed and guidance for MV interventions is lacking. Pressure loading in static exercise and volume loading with dynamic exercise can result in increasing LV volumes ventricular dilation and altered MV geometry, even in the absence of volume changes.[4]

A significant increase in EROA during semi-supine exercise (defined as an increase by greater than >13 mm) was shown to be associated with similar mortality rates and HF hospitalizations as severe secondary MR at rest.[15] Per ASE guidelines, an increased PA pressure during exercise (>60 mm Hg) "may be" important in asymptomatic severe primary MR.[11] Exercise right heart catheterization (RHC) can be particularly useful in identifying patients who are symptomatic due to mitral regurgitation that worsens with exercise and whose resting hemodynamics or echocardiogram do not support severe MR.[16]

MEDICAL MANAGEMENT OF FUNCTIONAL MITRAL REGURGITATION

Aggressive guideline-directed heart failure medical therapy (GDMT) can effectively reduce ventricular-functional MR by facilitating reverse remodeling and volume reduction of the LV and remains the backbone of FMR treatment.[13] The degree of FMR in both ischemic and nonischemic cardiomyopathies can be reduced by 28% to 50% this way.[17,18] In a single-center retrospective study of patients with at least 3+ FMR, 27% of patients evaluated for MV intervention achieved at least a 1 grade reduction in mitral regurgitation with medical therapy. Responders had smaller LV sizes, shorter QRS durations, and lower EROA/LVEDV ratios and more frequently received angiotensin-converting enzyme inhibitor (ACE-I) or angiotensin receptor/neprilysin inhibitors (ARNIs). In contrast, 18% of patients with nonsevere MR progressed to severe MR during the median follow-up period of 50 months despite maximal doses of GDMT, demonstrating a subset of patients with valvular disease that do not respond to medical therapy.[18] It is this phenotype of the nonresponder to GDMT that are most likely to benefit from mitral valvular interventions. In fact, it is hypothesized that one of the main differentiators between the very positive COAPT (Cardiovascular Outcomes Assessment of the MitraClip Percutaneous Therapy for Heart Failure Patients with Functional Mitral Regurgitation) trial and neutral MITRA-FR (Percutaneous Repair with the MitraClip Device for Severe Functional/Secondary Mitral Regurgitation) trial was the degree of optimization. The COAPT trial had stringent optimization requirements including an eligibility committee that confirmed the use of maximal doses of GDMT.[19] However, the MITRA-FR trial just required the participants to be on optimal standard of care therapy for HF according to investigator.[20]

The most contemporary heart failure GDMT relies on 4 key classes of medications. For patients with NYHA class II/III HFrEF (LVEF <40%), there is a class IA recommendation for renin-angiotensin-aldosterone blockade with an ACE-I or preferably ARNI if tolerated given results from the PARADIGM-HF trial showing superiority compared with ACE-I in reduction of the composite endpoint of HF hospitalization and cardiovascular (CV) death.[21] Use of bisoprolol, sustained-release metoprolol succinate, or carvedilol for neurohormonal blockade are also a Class IA recommendation, as are mineralocorticoid receptor antagonists (MRA), including spironolactone or eplerenone and sodium-glucose cotransporter 2 inhibitors (SGLT2is; Class IA).[22] Although conventionally GDMT was previously initiated in a sequential manner, a more aggressive approach is feasible and associated with improved outcomes.[23] The authors from STRONG-HF documented the superiority of rapid uptitration of GDMT coupled with close outpatient follow-up and its effect on reducing symptom burden, overall mortality and HF-related readmissions.[24]

The specific effects of individual classes of medications on FMR have been selectively investigated. In an early randomized controlled trial (RCT) in New York Heart Association (NYHA) class II/III HF with at least 2+ FMR, captopril, led to significant reductions in mitral regurgitant area, accompanied by improvement in stroke volume and reduction in systemic vascular resistance and left atrial area during a 12-week period.[25] More recently, the PRIME trial (Pharmacologic Reduction of Functional, Ischemic Mitral Regurgitation) showed a greater reduction in EROA, and LV diastolic volumes with ARNI compared with losartan in patients with FMR.[26] In addition to facilitating reverse modeling, ARNIs reduce preload and afterload, and inhibit tissue growth factor, which can cause leaflet thickening.[17] Although their beneficial effect on reverse remodeling, HF hospitalizations, and mortality are clear and reflected in current HF guidelines,[22] there is currently no direct evidence yet for SGLT2is and MRA's impact on FMR.

Among beta blockers, carvedilol has been shown to reduce RVol, EROA, and the FMR jet area.[27,28] The greatest extent of LV reverse remodeling has been found in patients in whom FMR improved, further confirming that FMR in itself can propagate disadvantageous remodeling, not just vice versa.[29,30]

Optimization in the modern era of cardiomyopathy is a complex and time-intensive process that requires frequent medication titration and follow-up (Fig. 1). Prognostication and trajectory of the cardiomyopathy is not able to be determined until they are optimized both

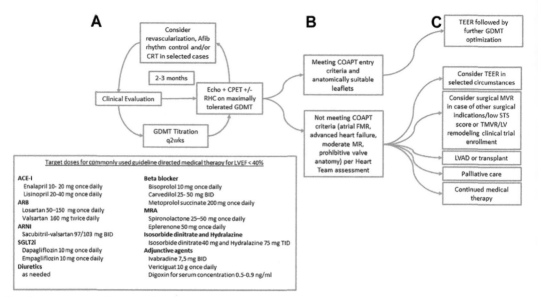

Fig. 1. Optimization clinic paradigm for FMR: (*A*) GDMT uptitration to maximum doses achieved in clinical trials or maximally tolerated doses within a 2 to 3 months' time frame followed by clinical reassessment and HF staging procedures including CPET and/or RHC and (*B*) Consideration for additional therapies including CRT, atrial fibrillation rhythm control, coronary revascularization. (*C*) In case of persistent, symptomatic, at least 3+ mitral regurgitation, comprehensive heart team assessment regarding suitability for MV interventions or other surgical HF therapies. CPET, cardiopulmonary exercise testing; CRT, cardiac resynchronization therapy; FMR, functional mitral regurgitation; GDMT, guideline directed medical therapy; RHC, right heart catheterization; TEER, transcatheter edge-to-edge repair.

pharmacologically and nonpharmacologically. Unfortunately—as experienced in GUIDE-IT—only a fraction of eligible HF patients ends up on truly maximally tolerated medical therapy even within the framework of a clinical HF trial.[31] The 2020 ACC/AHA valve and 2022 ACC/AHA HF guidelines therefore both emphasize the need for a multidisciplinary team conducting the medical optimization before consideration of any invasive options.[13]

In selected patients with a left bundle-branch block, particularly when the QRS duration exceeds 150 milliseconds, CRT has been shown to reduce FMR acutely and chronically, improve quality of life and hemodynamic profile in patients with persistently depressed systolic function and symptom burden despite maximally tolerated GDMT.[32] Intraventricular and interventricular synchronization resulting in increased cardiac output and reduced LV filling pressures in addition to sympatho-inhibitory effects resulting in a reversal of skeletal myopathy are among the mechanisms at play. Those who continue to have at least moderate-to-severe MR 3 months after CRT and despite optimized volume and afterload—which might require verification through invasive hemodynamics in selected patients—are suitable for a referral to the multidisciplinary valve team for the evaluation for MV

therapies. Unsurprisingly, the persistence of moderate-to-severe FMR after CRT has been shown to be a negative prognostic factor with increased mortality.[33] In the PERMIT-CARE registry, 51 patients who remained symptomatic (NYHA III–IV) with significant FMR (grade ≥2) post-CRT still derived improvement in functional class, left ventricular ejection fraction (LVEF) and reduction in LV volumes with transcatheter edge-to-edge repair (TEER).[34] In contrast to CRT, the role of coronary revascularization in the management of FMR is less clear even when evaluated appropriately in those with FMR secondary to ischemic heart disease. In a study of 136 patients with ischemic moderate MR, for example, 40% of patients continued to have functional MR after coronary artery bypass graft surgery.[35] Of 137 patients with severe ischemic MR, following percutaneous coronary intervention, a third of patients had improvement in their MR with an additional 29% requiring additional intervention.[36] Careful assessment of the mechanism of FMR would be key before pursuing revascularization.

It is possible to achieve a wide range of outcomes with optimization of cardiomyopathy using modern pharmacologic and device-based therapies. This can include everything from total myocardial recovery to end-stage/advanced HF requiring transplantation/left ventricular assist device (LVAD).[37] With optimization, we are frequently able to observe myocardial recovery or at least improvement to a point where advanced therapies such as LVAD or transplant can be avoided or delayed. Transcatheter intervention of FMR plays a pivotal role in optimization of cardiomyopathy and, in some cases, can also delay or completely avoid advanced therapies.

Atrial Functional Mitral Regurgitation

The ideal management for AFMR remains an area of investigation but theoretically medications that reverse LA remodeling should be used.[38] In a Phase 2 randomized clinical trial of patients with HFpEF (PARAMOUNT), sacubitril-valsartan reduced LA size primarily in patients without AF, however, did not demonstrate a significant reduction in atrial FMR.[39] In PARAGON-HF, the subgroup of patients deriving most benefit were women, patients with AF, and those with EF 57% or lesser, possibly mediated by a reduction of MR severity, although not explicitly assessed.[40] Despite the robust evidence regarding cardiac remodeling and CV outcomes for SGLT2 inhibitors and spironolactone in patients with heart failure independent of ejection fraction, their specific effects on atrial FMR have not been examined to date.

A recent HFpEF JACC scientific statement highlights the role of those 3 agents reducing mortality and HF hospitalizations among patients with HFpEF but the direct impact on AFMR remains to be seen.[41]

In regard to AF, both ablation and cardioversion when successful have been associated with reduced MR.[42] TEE evaluation of 43 patients after successful catheter ablation for persistent AF demonstrated reduction in the degree of MR and mitral annulus area in both anterior-posterior and medial-lateral directions, as well as improved mitral annular contraction.[43] Targeting rhythm control is one of the key interventions in this subgroup.[6]

LIMITED DATA FOR SURGICAL MITRAL VALVE REPAIR OR REPLACEMENT

According to the latest 2021 European Society of Cardiology/European Association for Cardio-Thoracic Surgery (ESC/EACTS) guidelines for the management of valvular heart disease,[14] there is a class I recommendation for "valve surgery/intervention" in patients with severe secondary MR who are symptomatic despite GDMT and CRT if indicated. A key point is that the decision should be decided by a "structured collaborative Heart Team." Data from randomized trials comparing mitral-valve surgery with medical therapy or transcatheter therapy in patients with FMR are unfortunately lacking.

In an analysis of 261 patients who underwent mitral annuloplasty and coronary revascularization for moderate-to-severe, functional MR, there was a low rate of recurrent MR after 10 years of follow-up.[44] In comparison to MV repair, chordal sparing MV replacement showed no significant difference in mortality or rates of LV reverse remodeling.[45]

Current American Heart Association/American College of Cardiology (AHA/ACC) guidelines recommend MV surgery in class IIA for patients with FMR undergoing concomitant bypass or aortic valve surgery and in class IIB for patients with persistent symptoms (NYHA class III–IV) despite optimal medical therapy, considering it reasonable to choose chordal-sparing MV replacement over repair. Due to inconsistent benefit and elevated surgical risk, isolated valve surgery is uncommonly performed for FMR, and if a surgical option is required, transplantation or LVAD therapy is often pursued.[5,46]

USE OF TRANSCATHETER EDGE-TO-EDGE REPAIR FOR PERCUTANEOUS MITRAL VALVE REPAIR

Percutaneous MV repair using a TEER has been proposed to correct FMR because this offers the potential for a less-invasive, lower risk alternative to surgical repair or replacement. TEER of the MV is performed via femoral transvenous and transseptal access using a platform that under TEE guidance deploys a clip, which grasps the anterior and posterior leaflets, resulting in an Alfieri stitch type repair and a resultant double-barrel orifice. As surgical MV repair or replacement has been effective in primary degenerative MR, TEER was first investigated in this population and found to be safe and effective.[47,48] Its utility was next evaluated in functional MR. Given that surgical MV repair has not led to a similar improvement in outcomes, it was unclear whether TEER would provide benefit to patients with FMR despite optimal GDMT.[45,49] However, in 2019, the first TEER platform received Food and Drug Administration approval for patients with at least moderate-to-severe FMR based on the results of pivotal clinical trials using the MitraClip device (Abbott Vascular: Santa Clara, CA, USA).[50] The MitraClip device was first studied, being used in 2 prospective clinical trials: COAPT and MITRA-FR.[19,20] Interestingly COAPT showed a significantly lower rate of all-cause mortality as well as a lower rate of HF hospitalizations at 2 years compared with medical therapy, whereas MITRA-FR did not show significant differences at 1 year. Detailed analysis of the 2 populations led to a possible explanation for this discrepancy in outcomes.

First, the inclusion criteria differed with the COAPT trial including those with more severe MR–EROA greater than 30 mm² and RVol greater than 45 mL, compared with MITRA-FR including those with EROA greater than 20 mm² and RVol greater than 30 mL. COAPT also aimed to include those with less severe LV and RV dysfunction as evidenced by LV ejection fraction of 20% to 50% (vs 15%–40%), LV end systolic diameter less than 70 mm (vs no limit on LV end systolic diameter), and exclusion of those with pulmonary artery systolic pressure greater than 70 mm Hg and moderate-severe RV systolic dysfunction (vs no RV function criteria in MITRA-FR). These led to the baseline characteristics differing with a higher mean EROA, lower LV end diastolic volume, and lower systolic pulmonary artery pressure in COAPT. The COAPT population was likely truly refractory to maximum medical therapy given that patients were excluded before randomization if they showed improvement in symptoms or degree of MR during the run-in period. This resulted in less patients with NYHA class I or II symptoms and higher N-terminal pro-B-type natriuretic peptide levels. Second, the procedural safety and efficacy differed with MitraClip procedural success of 95% in COAPT versus 91% in MITRA-FR. As a result, at 1 year approximately 10% fewer subjects in COAPT were found to have grade 2 MR or greater severity compared with MITRA-FR.

Based on these data, the 2020 ACC/AHA guidelines for valvular heart disease and 2022 ACC/AHA/HFSA guidelines for HF provide a class IIA recommendation to consider TEER for patients with LV EF less than 50% and at least 3+ FMR who have refractory symptoms despite maximum medical therapy in addition to LV end systolic diameter less than 70 mm and pulmonary artery systolic pressure less than 70 mm Hg.[13] Only if their anatomy is not favorable should they be referred for consideration of surgical MV replacement. These recommendations were further supported by the publication of the 5-year results of COAPT.[51] There was a 10% absolute risk reduction in all-cause mortality and an 18% absolute risk reduction in death or HF hospitalization (hazard ratio 0.53 (95% CI, 0.44–0.64). Safety was also demonstrated with device-specific safety events occurring in only 1.4% of the 293 patients, all within 30 days of the procedure. The most recent generation, the MitraClip G4, is under investigation in the EXPAND G4 trial with promising preliminary results. The G4 device is available in 4 sizes with combinations of 2 different arm lengths (12 mm for XT/XTW and 9 mm for NT/NTW) and widths (4 mm for NT/XT and 6 mm for NTW/XTW).[52]

An alternative TEER device was introduced known as the PASCAL system (Edwards Lifesciences, CA, USA), which aimed to address limitations found in the earlier generations of MitraClip such as inadequate MR reduction and leaflet injury.[53,54] The key new features of the PASCAL system included wider paddles and arms that are made of a more elastic ninitol-based system to approximate the leaflets. The PASCAL system also allows independent leaflet grasping. Its retention system is horizontally arranged at the distal edge of the clasps, compared with longitudinally along the grippers in the MitraClip system. A prospective trial (NCT03706833) comparing the PASCAL and MitraClip systems was designed known as the CLASP IID (for degenerative MR) and CLASP IIF (for FMR).[48] CLASP IID demonstrated the PASCAL system to be noninferior to MitraClip for degenerative MR. By the time of completion of the study, there were subsequent iterations of the MitraClip design with the fourth generation (G4) system addressing earlier concerns. The results of the CLASP IIF trial are currently awaited. The Pascal device has 2 sizes, the original and the narrower Ace implant (10-mm vs 6-mm paddles).

Additional trials have been designed and completed to evaluate TEER in FMR (Table 1). The RESHAPE-HF2 (A Clinical Evaluation of the Safety and Effectiveness of the MitraClip System in the Treatment of Clinically Significant Functional Mitral Regurgitation) trial is a prospective single-arm trial to evaluate the MitraClip system with the primary outcome being composite rate of recurrent HF hospitalizations and CV death at 2 years.[55] Real-world experience from prospective registries is encouraging as well. Society of Thoracic Surgeons/American College of Cardiology Transcatheter Valve Therapy (STS/ACC TVT) registry data showed that the number of patients receiving TEER who had FMR increased to 1576 in 2019. Among those 7.5% had greater than moderate, residual MR and 1.2% required reintervention at 30 days. This resulted in the majority of patients (76.7%) improving to NYHA functional class I or II and overall Kansas City Cardiomyopathy Questionnaire (KCCQ) quality of life score improving by approximately 30 points at the 30-day follow-up.[56] The

Table 1
Completed and currently enrolling randomized controlled trials for transcatheter edge-to-edge repair in functional mitral regurgitation

	COAPT	MITRA-FR	RESHAPE-HF2	MITRADVANCE-HF	MATTERHORN
Status of trial	Completed Results published	Completed Results published	Recruiting	Recruiting	Recruiting
LVEF	20%–50% (and LV end systolic diameter $\leq$ 70 mm)	15%–40%	15%–35% (NYHA class II) 15%–45% (NYHA class III/IV)	$\leq$35%	$\geq$20%
MR severity	Grade 3+ or 4+	EROA >20 mm^2 and/ or RVol >30 mL	Moderate-severe or severe MR (EROA $\geq$30 mm^2)	EROA $\geq$30 mm^2	Clinically significant MR
Intervention being studied	MitraClip vs optimal medical therapy	MitraClip vs optimal medical therapy	MitraClip vs optimal medical therapy	MitraClip vs optimal medical therapy	MitraClip vs MV surgery
Primary outcome	Cumulative HF hospitalization at 2 y	Death and HF hospitalization at 1 y	Composite rate of recurrent HF hospitalizations and cardiovascular death	Absolute change in overall KCCQ summary score (KCCQ-OS) at 3 mo	Composite of death, rehospitalization for HF, reintervention, assist device implantation and stroke at 12 mo after intervention
Number of subjects	614	304	650 (estimated)	172 (estimated)	210 (estimated)

MitraClip Global Expand registry is a prospective observational postmarketing study of 1041 patients who received the MitraClip for 3+ or 4+ symptomatic MR across 57 site and 7 countries, of which 413 subjects were deemed to have functional MR based on core-laboratory analysis.[57] This showed a sustained reduction in MR severity with 93% of patients deemed to have 1+ MR or lesser at 1 year.

TEER shows promise for treatment of FMR; however, patient selection, favorable anatomic consideration, and optimization of GDMT seem to be keys to ongoing further success.

PATIENT SELECTION: THE OPTIMAL TIMING, HEMODYNAMIC PHENOTYPING, AND RISK STRATIFICATION

The optimal timing for TEER remains poorly defined and the procedural success is highly dependent on patient selection. Hence, clinical, functional, and multimodality imaging assessment of the patient should be part of a comprehensive and meticulous workup to help direct the clinicians to those patients who could derive the maximal benefit from TEER. Patients who have not been optimized medically or patients who remain minimally symptomatic are less likely to benefit from MV repair. Truly advanced patients with HF beyond COAPT inclusion criteria (ambulatory NYHA class IV) are most likely better served with surgical advanced HF therapies including cardiac transplantation or LVAD, although there might be an indication overlap in patients with the Interagency Registry for Mechanically Assisted Circulatory Support (INTERMACS) profiles 4 to 6 and some patients might not be candidates for surgical advanced HF therapies (Table 2 and Fig. 2)

RHC can be helpful in selected cases to define intracardiac hemodynamics including the degree of pulmonary hypertension, provide HF staging, and prognostic information, especially if it is difficult to tease out functional impairment by clinical history alone. Additionally, cardiopulmonary exercise testing (CPET) can provide incremental information regarding cardiovascular reserve capacity and functional class, dynamic mitral regurgitation, HF prognosis, and potential candidacy for truly advanced HF therapies.[59,60] A peak VO_2 value of 10 mL/kg/min was identified as the best cutoff for prediction of cardiac and all-cause death and HF hospitalization in this severe FMR population.[61] Other gas exchange parameters being used for prognostication include ventilatory efficiency (VE/VCO$_2$ slope), circulatory power (peak oxygen consumption × peak systolic blood pressure, presence of exercise oscillatory ventilation, abnormal oxygen uptake efficiency slope, and heart rate recovery. Their additive prognostic value can be used in commonly available risk scores.[62] Some of these more advanced patients with HF might delay need for cardiac transplant or could respond to a point not needing cardiac transplant any longer. On the other side, even the device arm of the medically optimized COAPT randomized control trial reported a 57% mortality 5 years after device placement[51]; hence, these patients benefit from longitudinal management by a multidisciplinary team including an HF specialist.

Procedural outcomes and effect on LV systolic function can help to risk stratify patients after TEER. Acute reduction in LVEF is not uncommon after TEER, is associated with worse outcomes, and can be partially explained by the rapid increase in LV afterload, related to the rapid loss of the low-resistance "shunt" into the left atrium.[63] Additionally, procedural success defined by mild MR (or less) and/or mean left atrial pressure of less than 15 after Clip(s) placement can be a very powerful prognosticator for 1 year survival and could help triaging patients to alternative therapies postprocedure.[2]

Of note, some ambulatory class IV patient with HF might not be considered candidates for surgical advanced HF therapy temporarily. Data from the MitraBridge registry provides reassuring results and rationale to consider TEER even in this situation. In 153 class IV patients with HF, who were either listed for cardiac transplant or currently not considered candidate for such, the majority of patients were able to become eligible for transplant listing, received a heart transplant, or even became well enough not to require heart transplant any longer during a time period of 2 years.[64]

PATIENT SELECTION: CLINICAL CONSIDERATIONS
Independent Risk Factors
The sole assessment of baseline MV anatomy and LV morphology does not accurately predict the outcome before and/or after TEER. In COAPT patients with NYHA functional classes II, III, and ambulatory IV at baseline all benefited clinically from MitraClip therapy, however, higher baseline NYHA functional class was strongly associated with a greater risk for adverse events with or without TEER. A 28% higher risk of mortality or HF hospitalizations per 1 NYHA class increase was noted in COAPT at 2 years.[65] Hence, surgical advanced HF therapies in the form of cardiac

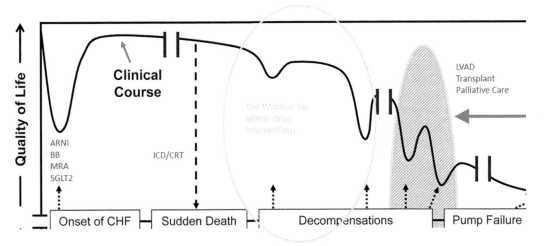

Fig. 2. Optimal timing of edge-to-edge MV interventions.[58] (*Adapter from* Allen LA, Stevenson LW, Grady KL, Goldstein NE, Matlock DD, Arnold RM, et al. Decision making in advanced heart failure: a scientific statement from the American Heart Association. Circulation. 2012;125(15):1928 to 52.)

transplant or LVAD should be at least considered for ambulatory class IV patients with HF—either alternatively or sequentially. It is noteworthy that after edge-to-edge repair and the associated increase in transmitral gradients LVAD might become a less-attractive option downstream, which becomes relevant in scenarios where transplant is not an option at all.

Several parameters affected by abnormal right ventricular contractility and right ventricular afterload (RV–PA coupling) serve as important prognosticator for postprocedural outcomes, in particular significant tricuspid regurgitation.[66] Moreover, in COAPT, MitraClip reduced 30-day PA systolic pressures and 2-year rates of death or HFH compared with GDMT alone, irrespective of baseline pulmonary artery systolic pressure (PASP). However, elevated PASPs are

associated with a worse prognosis in patients with FMR. Similarly, advanced RV dysfunction as assessed by RV–PA uncoupling is an additional powerful predictor of 2-year adverse outcomes in patients with FMR and should be part of the clinical decision-making and prognostication.[67,68] Despite similar rates of procedural success (>90%), patients with RV dysfunction (TAPSE $\leq$16 mm) are less likely to derive a clinical benefit from Mitraclip in terms of functional capacity and survival than patients with normal RV function (TAPSE >16 mm).[69]

MitraClip registry data are able to provide additional clues on how to identify higher risk patients. These include patients with more advanced renal disease, very low ejection fraction, and chronic obstructive pulmonary disease (COPD).[70,71] Overall anatomic and clinical risk assessment can

Table 2
Functional class phenotypes and their relationship to transcatheter edge-to-edge repair candidacy

INTERMACS Profiles	Objective Criteria	Official Shorthand	NYHA Class Equivalent
INTERMACS level 1	Cardiac index <2.2	"Crash and burn"	IV
INTERMACS level 2	Cardiac index <2.2	"Sliding fast"	IV
INTERMACS level 3	Cardiac index <2.2	Inotrope dependent	IV
INTERMACS level 4	Peak VO2 < 12	Resting symptoms	Amb IV [a]
INTERMACS level 5	Peak VO2 < 12	"Housebound"	Amb IV [a]
INTERMACS level 6		"Walking wounded"	IIIB [a]
INTERMACS level 7		Advanced class III	III [a]

INTERMACS levels 4–7 consistent with favorable "COAPT phenotype," positive registry signals for selected patients INTERMACS 2–3
[a] Included in COAPT.

provide additional guidance toward TEER, advanced HF therapies, or potential futility.

In select cases, cardiac MRI is able to provide MR quantification in case of suboptimal echocardiographic images or discordant imaging and/or clinical findings. Additionally, the quantification of scar burden (myocardial infarct size) can provide incremental prognostic information in patient with underlying ischemic cardiomyopathy and ischemic MR.[72]

Red Flags Favoring Surgical, Advanced Heart Failure Therapies over Transcatheter Edge-To-Edge Repair

In the absence of objective data obtained through RHC and CPET, there are other clinical clues helping to identify end-stage patients with HF and the need for more advanced HF therapies. These includes include refractory NYHA class 3B of 4 HF symptoms, frequent HF-related hospitalizations, worsening hyponatremia and cardiorenal syndrome, increasing diuretic requirements and inability to tolerate meaningful neurohormonal blockade, frequent ventricular arrhythmias, cardiac cachexia, or high mortality risk from validated risk predictor models (eg, Seattle heart failure model).[73,74]

PATIENT SELECTION: ANATOMICAL CONSIDERATIONS

In light of the discrepant results of the MITRA-FR and COAPT trials, which ultimately influenced contemporary guidelines, it seems reasonable to conclude that the MitraClip procedure reduces HF hospitalization and mortality in patients meeting the following characteristics.

1. Moderate-to-severe or greater secondary MR defined as EROA $\geq$30 mm^2 and/or RVol >45 mL;
2. LVEF between 20% and 50% and LV end-systolic diameter less than 70 mm;
3. Persistent HF symptoms (NYHA $\geq$ II) despite optimal (maximally tolerated) GDMT with CRT and coronary revascularization if appropriate.
4. Absence of severe pulmonary hypertension (PASP >70 mm Hg) and/or severe right ventricular dysfunction.

Furthermore, the goal of the procedure should be to obtain an acute reduction of the MR severity to mild or lesser and the implantation of additional clips should be considered to achieve this goal. In a real-world cohort of patients with FMR undergoing TEER, the retrospective application of adapted COAPT enrollment criteria successfully identified

a specific phenotype demonstrating lower mortality rates. On the contrary, stratification according to adapted MITRA-FR criteria resulted in comparable outcomes.[75]

Some authors recently presented at conceptual framework delineating 2 major profiles of significant secondary MR:[76]

a. disproportionate" MR referring to an RVol disproportionately higher than the degree of LV dilatation. Such patients are likely to mainly benefit from a therapy targeted to the MV with TEER, beyond GDMT and/or CRT.
b. proportionate" MR refers to an RVol proportional to the degree of LV remodeling. This group would likely benefit the most from strategies aimed at reducing LV size alone, not directed to MV apparatus.

Proportionate MR is designated by an EROA (mm^2)/LVEDV (mL) ratio of roughly less than 0.15. From this viewpoint, most patients enrolled in MITRA-FR would have proportionate MR, where mean LVEDV and EROA were 252 mL and 31 mm^2, respectively. Conversely, subjects included in COAPT trial had LVEDV 30% smaller (mean 192 mL) and EROA 30% larger (mean 41 mm^2) than MITRA-FR patients, and MR seemed to be far "out of context" to the degree of LV disease. The small group of patients in the COAPT trial who had the features of proportionate MR and were similar to those enrolled in the MITRA-FR trial did not respond favorably to TEER. However, other recently published post hoc secondary analysis of both trials suggest that the proportionate-disproportionate hypothesis alone may not be enough to explain the divergent results of MITRA-FR and COAPT.

Beyond determining the "proportionality" of the regurgitant yet related to the degree of LV remodeling, TEE imaging remains key for preprocedural planning and determining candidacy for TEER.

Other important structures to interrogate are interatrial septum (and its suitability for septal puncture), concomitant right ventricular dimensions and function, concomitant tricuspid regurgitation, estimated pulmonary artery pressure, leaflet length and calcifications within the planned grasping zone, as well as baseline transmitral gradients (Fig. 3).

Of note, the decision-making in atrial FMR remains less defined despite emerging registry data suggesting atrial reverse remodeling and symptom improvement after TEER.[77] Current ACC/AHA guidelines provide a class 2b (LOE B) recommendation in this situation.[13]

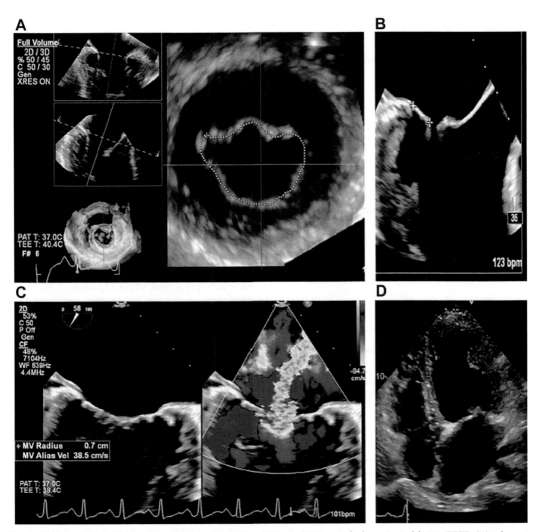

Fig. 3. TTE study in a patient presenting with functional MR and MV morphology "suitable" to TEER: (A) adequate MVA (>4 cm^2); (B) posterior leaflet mobile length ≥10 mm; (C) symmetric tethering of noncalcified leaflets with central regurgitant jet; and (D) preserved leaflet coaptation. MR, mitral regurgitation; MVA, mitral valve area; TEER, transcatheter edge-to-edge repair; TTE, transthoracic echocardiography.

FUTURE DIRECTIONS: EXPANDING CRITERIA

The clinical landscape is evolving quickly since MITRA-FR and COAPT were published in 2018. The 2022 HF guidelines now include novel agents as part of the quadruple therapy with an enhanced mortality benefit with GDMT only. On the other side, the new device generations (Mitraclip G4 and PASCAL) have advanced technically and are more likely to result in postprocedural MR reduction. Therefore, indications and timing for TEER over GDMT alone will require further fine tuning in the current era. Real-word clinical experience and outcomes associated with the use of the newer generation MitraClip systems have

been recently reported of part of the ongoing EXPAND Study. The study documented a high proportion of patients with FMR are currently being treated outside COAPT eligibility criteria. New generation devices have higher percent of patients with MR reduction to mild, compared to first-generation device used in COAPT. No subjects in either non-COAPT like group (moderate MR and advanced HF) experienced residual MR greater than 3+ at the 1-year follow-up. Longer term follow-up of these patients and comparison with patients treated with GDMT only will be important to determine the impact of MitraClip on their outcomes in moderate MR, exercise-induced MR, or in advanced HF.[78] According to the same registry, even NYHA class IV patients can benefit through a significant

Table 3
Patient selection summary relying on anatomic, clinical, and heart failure staging components

Determinants of Edge-To-Edge Mitral Valve Repair Efficacy in Functional Mitral Regurgitation	
Optimal	**Unsuitable**
NYHA class II–IVa	Asymptomatic or advanced, stage D HF beyond ambulatory NYHA class IV
MV area >4 cm^2	MV area <3 cm^2, mean gradient >5 mm Hg
Disproportionate mitral regurgitation (EROA/LVEDV ratio >0.14)	Disproportionate LV remodeling (LVEF <20% and/or LVESD >7 cm)
Posterior leaflet length >10 mm	Posterior leaflet length <7 mm and/or coaptation depth >11 mm
Normal right ventricular function and transpulmonary gradients	Severe right ventricular dysfunction and/or irreversible pulmonary hypertension (systolic PA pressures > 70 mm Hg)
	Significant scar burden on cardiac MRI
Low-risk CPET	High-risk CPET (VO$_2$ peak < 14 mL/kg/min or < 50% predicted, VE/VCO$_2$ slope > 36, oscillatory ventilation, hypotensive response to exercise)
No leaflet calcifications	Significant leaflet calcifications at grasping area
Coaptation depth <11 mm, coaptation length >2 mm	Need for non-MR–related cardiac surgery
On maximally tolerated HF medical regimen according to 2022 ACC/AHA guidelines	COPD requiring oxygen or steroids
No residual coronary ischemia	History of or active endocarditis or rheumatic heart diseases

improvement in functional class improvement after TEER.[79] European guidelines recommend the consideration of TEER even in patients who do not fulfill the COAPT criteria but in whom TEER may improve symptoms and quality of life (class IIb) or as a bridge to surgical, advanced HF therapies.[80]

Registry data (STS/ACC TVT Registry) including 1044 cases of FMR also report the feasibility and associated mortality reduction of TEER in the setting of cardiogenic shock as a bridge to more permanent therapies.[81] Procedural success was defined as final MR grade < 2+ (occurred in 88.2%) and MR reduction > 1 grade (occurred in 91.4%). HF readmission rates and mortality were significantly lower in those with a successful procedure (29.6% vs 45.2%; 95% CI 0.42–0.62). A confirmatory RCT is currently ongoing.[82]

FUTURE DIRECTIONS: NEW DEVICE PLATFORMS

Although the newer generation of available TEER devices and procedural advancements has expanded the range of patients currently eligible for such, multiple other minimally invasive transcatheter therapies are under investigation to further safely and effectively treat FMR patients. For example, the TWIST-EFS trial for the Innovalve System (Innovalve Bio Medical: Tel Hashomer – Ramat Gan, Israel), the SUMMIT trial for the Tendyne device (Abbott), and the APPOLO trial for the Intrepid device (Medtronic: Minneapolis, MN, USA) are all ongoing trials for transcatheter MV replacement devices. The Carillon Mitral Contour System (Cardiac Dimensions), currently under investigation in the EMPOWER trial, simulates a surgical ring annuloplasty by inserting a transcatheter device through the coronary sinus. Some of these transcather MV replacement platforms have to potential to overcome anatomic limitations precluding the use of TEER in a subset of patient.[83]

SUMMARY

In summary, the sole assessment of baseline MV anatomy and LV morphology does not accurately predict the outcome before and after TEER. Other relevant comorbidities and HF stage/functional class will influence therapeutic decision making, which requires a thoughtful approach carried out through a multidisciplinary compromising of HF specialists, imaging physicians, interventionalists, surgeons, and electrophysiologists (Table 3). Current ACC/AHA heart failure and valve guidelines provide guidance on how to optimize patients with FMR before any MV interventions and how to triage them to TEER, surgical MV replacement, percutaneous MV replacement clinic trials or even truly advanced HF therapies. In some cases, this heart team can turn patients from a MITRA-FR phenotype with some degree of "pre-habing" to a COAPT phenotype with more favorable right ventricular hemodynamics and periprocedural outcomes. Most patients can benefit from a heart team-guided "rehabing" postprocedure by adjusting their GDMT to capture the best possible outcomes.[66]

CLINICS CARE POINTS

- The inclusion criteria of the landmark COAPT clinical trial define a patient subset most likely to benefit from transcatheter mitral edge-to-edge repair.

- Hemodynamic phenotyping in the form of RHC and CPET can unmask stage D HF stages more likely to benefit from surgical advanced HF therapies.

- Immediate response to transcatheter mitral edge-to-edge repair in the form of mitral regurgitation reduction, reduction of left atrial pressures, and favorable response of systolic function can predict the patient's trajectory postprocedure and need for alternative, therapies.

DECLARATION OF INTERESTS

Authors have no conflict of interest to declare.

REFERENCES

1. Varadarajan P, Sharma S, Heywood JT, et al. High prevalence of clinically silent severe mitral regurgitation in patients with heart failure: role for echocardiography. J Am Soc Echocardiogr 2006;19(12):1458–61.
2. Bartko PE, Heitzinger G, Pavo N, et al. Burden, treatment use, and outcome of secondary mitral regurgitation across the spectrum of heart failure: observational cohort study. BMJ 2021;373:n1421.
3. Karagodin I, Singh A, Lang RM. Pathoanatomy of mitral regurgitation. Struct Heart 2020;4(4):254–63.
4. Bertrand PB, Schwammenthal E, Levine RA, et al. Exercise dynamics in secondary mitral regurgitation: pathophysiology and therapeutic implications. Circulation 2017;135(3):297–314.
5. Coats AJS, Anker SD, Baumbach A, et al. The management of secondary mitral regurgitation in patients with heart failure: a joint position statement from the Heart Failure Association (HFA), European Association of Cardiovascular Imaging (EACVI), European Heart Rhythm Association (EHRA), and European Association of Percutaneous Cardiovascular Interventions (EAPCI) of the ESC. Eur Heart J 2021; 42(13):1254–69.
6. Reddy YNV, Nishimura RA. Not all secondary mitral regurgitation is the same-potential phenotypes and implications for mitral repair. JAMA Cardiol 2020;5(10):1087–8.
7. Bursi F, Enriquez-Sarano M, Jacobsen SJ, et al. Mitral regurgitation after myocardial infarction: a review. Am J Med 2006;119(2):103–12.
8. Zoghbi WA, Levine RA, Flachskampf F, et al. Atrial functional mitral regurgitation: a JACC: cardiovascular imaging expert panel viewpoint. JACC Cardiovasc Imaging 2022;15(11):1870–82.
9. Scholte AJ, Holman ER, Haverkamp MC, et al. Underestimation of severity of mitral regurgitation with varying hemodynamics. Eur J Echocardiogr 2005;6(4):297–300.
10. Grewal KS, Malkowski MJ, Piracha AR, et al. Effect of general anesthesia on the severity of mitral regurgitation by transesophageal echocardiography. Am J Cardiol 2000;85(2):199–203.
11. Zoghbi WA, Adams D, Bonow RO, et al. Recommendations for noninvasive evaluation of native valvular regurgitation: a report from the american society of echocardiography developed in collaboration with the society for cardiovascular magnetic resonance. J Am Soc Echocardiogr 2017;30(4): 303–71.
12. Faza NN, Chebrolu LB, El-Tallawi KC, et al. An integrative, multiparametric approach to mitral regurgitation evaluation: a case-based illustration. JACC Case Rep 2022;4(19):1231–41.
13. Otto CM, Nishimura RA, Bonow RO, et al. 2020 ACC/AHA guideline for the management of patients with valvular heart disease: a report of the american college of cardiology/american heart association joint committee on clinical practice guidelines. Circulation 2021;143(5):e72–227.
14. Vahanian A, Beyersdorf F, Praz F, et al, ESC/EACTS Scientific Document Group. 2021 ESC/EACTS guidelines for the management of valvular heart disease. Eur Heart J 2022;43(7):561–632.
15. Lancellotti P, Gerard PL, Pierard LA. Long-term outcome of patients with heart failure and dynamic functional mitral regurgitation. Eur Heart J 2005; 26(15):1528–32.
16. Valle FH, Mohammed B, Wright SP, et al. Exercise right heart catheterisation in cardiovascular

diseases: a guide to interpretation and consider-ations in the management of valvular heart disease. Interv Cardiol 2020;16:e01.

17. Milwidsky A, Mathai SV, Topilsky Y, et al. Medical therapy for functional mitral regurgitation. Circ Heart Fail 2022;15(9):e009689.

18. Sannino A, Sudhakaran S, Milligan G, et al. Effec-tiveness of medical therapy for functional mitral regurgitation in heart failure with reduced ejection fraction. J Am Coll Cardiol 2020;76(7):883–4.

19. Stone GW, Lindenfeld J, Abraham WT, et al, COAPT Investigators. Transcatheter mitral-valve repair in patients with heart failure. N Engl J Med 2018;379(24):2307–18.

20. Obadia JF, Messika-Zeitoun D, Leurent G, et al, MITRA-FR Investigators. Percutaneous repair or medical treatment for secondary mitral regurgita-tion. N Engl J Med 2018;379(24):2297–306.

21. McMurray JJ, Packer M, Desai AS, et al, PARA-DIGM-HF Investigators and Committees. Angio-tensin-neprilysin inhibition versus enalapril in heart failure. N Engl J Med 2014;371(11):993–1004.

22. Heidenreich PA, Bozkurt B, Aguilar D, et al. 2022 AHA/ACC/HFSA guideline for the management of heart failure: executive summary: a report of the american college of cardiology/american heart association joint committee on clinical practice guidelines. J Am Coll Cardiol 2022;79(17):1757–80.

23. McMurray JJV, Packer M. How should we sequence the treatments for heart failure and a reduced ejec-tion fraction?: a redefinition of evidence-based medicine. Circulation 2021;143(9):875–7.

24. Mebazaa A, Davison B, Chioncel O, et al. Safety, tolerability and efficacy of up-titration of guideline-directed medical therapies for acute heart failure (STRONG-HF): a multinational, open-label, randomised, trial. Lancet 2022;400(10367):1938–52.

25. Seneviratne B, Moore GA, West PD. Effect of captopril on functional mitral regurgitation in dilated heart failure: a randomised double blind placebo controlled trial. Br Heart J 1994;72(1):63–8.

26. Kang DH, Park SJ, Shin SH, et al. Angiotensin re-ceptor neprilysin inhibitor for functional mitral regurgitation. Circulation 2019;139(11):1354–65.

27. Capomolla S, Febo O, Gnemmi M, et al. Beta-blockade therapy in chronic heart failure: diastolic function and mitral regurgitation improvement by carvedilol. Am Heart J 2000;139(4):596–608.

28. Comin-Colet J, Sanchez-Corral MA, Manito N, et al. Effect of carvedilol therapy on functional mitral regurgitation, ventricular remodeling, and contractility in patients with heart failure due to left ventricular systolic dysfunction. Transplant Proc 2002;34(1):177–8.

29. Lowes BD, Gill EA, Abraham WT, et al. Effects of carvedilol on left ventricular mass, chamber geometry, and mitral regurgitation in chronic heart failure. Am J Cardiol 1999;83(8):1201–5.

30. Kotlyar E, Hayward CS, Keogh AM, et al. The impact of baseline left ventricular size and mitral regurgitation on reverse left ventricular remodel-ling in response to carvedilol: size doesn't matter. Heart 2004;90(7):800–1.

31. Fiuzat M, Ezekowitz J, Alemayehu W, et al. Assess-ment of limitations to optimization of guideline-directed medical therapy in heart failure from the guide-it trial: a secondary analysis of a randomized clinical trial. JAMA Cardiol 2020;5(7):757–64.

32. Parthenakis FI, Patrianakos AP, Simantirakis EN, et al. CRT and exercise capacity in heart failure: the impact of mitral valve regurgitation. Europace 2008;10(Suppl 3). iii96–100.

33. Spartera M, Galderisi M, Mele D, et al, Echocardio-graphic Study Group of the Italian Society of Cardi-ology SIC. Role of cardiac dyssynchrony and resynchronization therapy in functional mitral regur-gitation. Eur Heart J Cardiovasc Imaging 2016;17(5):471–80.

34. Auricchio A, Schillinger W, Meyer S, et al, PERMIT-CARE Investigators. Correction of mitral regurgita-tion in nonresponders to cardiac resynchronization therapy by MitraClip improves symptoms and pro-motes reverse remodeling. J Am Coll Cardiol 2011;58(21):2183–9.

35. Aklog L, Filsoufi F, Flores KQ, et al. Does coronary artery bypass grafting alone correct moderate ischemic mitral regurgitation? Circulation 2001;104(12 Suppl 1):I68–75.

36. Yousefzai R, Bajaj N, Krishnaswamy A, et al. Outcomes of patients with ischemic mitral regurgi-tation undergoing percutaneous coronary interven-tion. Am J Cardiol 2014;114(7):1011–7.

37. Rose EA, Gelijns AC, Moskowitz AJ, et al, Random-ized Evaluation of Mechanical Assistance for the Treatment of Congestive Heart Failure REMATCH Study Group. Long-term use of a left ventricular assist device for end-stage heart failure. N Engl J Med 2001;345(20):1435–43.

38. Deferm S, Bertrand PB, Verbrugge FH, et al. Atrial functional mitral regurgitation: JACC re-view topic of the week. J Am Coll Cardiol 2019;73(19):2465–76.

39. Solomon SD, Zile M, Pieske B, et al, Prospective comparison of ARNI with ARB on Management Of heart failUre with preserved ejectioN fracTion PARAMOUNT Investigators. The angiotensin re-ceptor neprilysin inhibitor LCZ696 in heart failure with preserved ejection fraction: a phase 2 double-blind randomised controlled trial. Lancet 2012;380(9851):1387–95.

40. Solomon SD, McMurray JJV, Anand IS, et al, PARAGON-HF Investigators and Committees. Angiotensin-Neprilysin inhibition in heart failure

with preserved ejection fraction. N Engl J Med 2019;381(17):1609–20.

41. Kittleson MM, Panjrath GS, Amancherla K, et al. 2023 ACC expert consensus decision pathway on management of heart failure with preserved ejection fraction: a report of the american college of cardiology solution set oversight committee. J Am Coll Cardiol 2023;81(18):1835–78.

42. Gertz ZM, Raina A, Saghy L, et al. Evidence of atrial functional mitral regurgitation due to atrial fibrillation: reversal with arrhythmia control. J Am Coll Cardiol 2011;58(14):1474–81.

43. Nishino S, Watanabe N, Ashikaga K, et al. Reverse remodeling of the mitral valve complex after radiofrequency catheter ablation for atrial fibrillation: a serial 3-dimensional echocardiographic study. Circ Cardiovasc Imaging 2019; 12(10):e009317.

44. Petrus AHJ, Dekkers OM, Tops LF, et al. Impact of recurrent mitral regurgitation after mitral valve repair for functional mitral regurgitation: long-term analysis of competing outcomes. Eur Heart J 2019;40(27):2206–14.

45. Goldstein D, Moskowitz AJ, Gelijns AC, et al, CTSN. Two-year outcomes of surgical treatment of severe ischemic mitral regurgitation. N Engl J Med 2016;374(4):344–53.

46. Mirabel M, Iung B, Baron G, et al. What are the characteristics of patients with severe, symptomatic, mitral regurgitation who are denied surgery? Eur Heart J 2007;28(11):1358–65.

47. Feldman T, Foster E, Glower DD, et al, EVEREST II Investigators. Percutaneous repair or surgery for mitral regurgitation. N Engl J Med 2011;364(15): 1395–406.

48. Lim DS, Smith RL, Gillam LD, et al, CLASP IID Pivotal Trial Investigators. Randomized Comparison of Transcatheter Edge-to-Edge Repair for Degenerative Mitral Regurgitation in Prohibitive Surgical Risk Patients. JACC Cardiovasc Interv 2022;15(24):2523–36.

49. Michler RE, Smith PK, Parides MK, et al, CTSN. Two-year outcomes of surgical treatment of moderate ischemic mitral regurgitation. N Engl J Med 2016;374(20):1932–41.

50. FDA approves new indication for valve repair device to treat certain heart failure patients with mitral regurgitation [Internet]. FDA. 2019, Available at: https://www.fda.gov/news-events/press-announcements/fda-approves-new-indication-valve-repair-device-treat-certain-heart-failure-patients-mitral.

51. Stone GW, Abraham WT, Lindenfeld J, et al, COAPT Investigators. Five-year follow-up after transcatheter repair of secondary mitral regurgitation. N Engl J Med 2023;388(22):2037–48.

52. von Bardeleben RS, Rogers JH, Mahoney P, et al. Real-world outcomes of fourth-generation mitral transcatheter repair: 30-day results From EXPAND G4. JACC Cardiovasc Interv 2023; 16(12):1463–73.

53. Asch FM, Little SH, Mackensen GB, et al. Incidence and standardised definitions of mitral valve leaflet adverse events after transcatheter mitral valve repair: the EXPAND study. EuroIntervention 2021; 17(11):e932–41.

54. Sugiura A, Kavsur R, Spieker M, et al. Recurrent mitral regurgitation after mitraclip: predictive factors, morphology, and clinical implication. Circ Cardiovasc Interv 2022;15(3):e010895.

55. Institut fuer anwendungsorientierte Forschung und klinische Studien Gmb H. A RandomizEd Study of tHe MitrACliP DEvice in Heart Failure Patients With Clinically Significant Functional Mitral Regurgitation [Internet]. 2021. Available at: https://clinicaltrials.gov/ct2/show/NCT02444338.

56. Mack M, Carroll JD, Thourani V, et al. Transcatheter mitral valve therapy in the united states: a report from the STS-ACC TVT registry. J Am Coll Cardiol 2021;78(23):2326–53.

57. Abbott Medical D. A Contemporary, Prospective Study Evaluating Real-world Experience of Performance and Safety for the Next Generation of MitraClip® Devices (EXPAND). Clinical trial registration. clinicaltrials.gov; 2021 2021/12/07/. Report No.: study/NCT03502811.

58. Allen LA, Stevenson LW, Grady KL, et al, American Heart Association, Council on Quality of Care and Outcomes Research, Council on Cardiovascular Nursing, Council on Clinical Cardiology, Council on Cardiovascular Radiology and Intervention, Council on Cardiovascular Surgery and Anesthesia. Decision making in advanced heart failure: a scientific statement from the American Heart Association. Circulation 2012;125(15):1928–52.

59. Hsu S, Fang JC, Borlaug BA. Hemodynamics for the heart failure clinician: a state-of-the-art review. J Card Fail 2022;28(1):133–48.

60. Malhotra R, Bakken K, D'Elia E, et al. Cardiopulmonary exercise testing in heart failure. JACC Heart Fail 2016;4(8):607–16.

61. Baldi C, Citro R, Silverio A, et al. Predictors of outcome in heart failure patients with severe functional mitral regurgitation undergoing MitraClip treatment. Int J Cardiol 2019;284:50–8.

62. Myers J, Arena R, Dewey F, et al. A cardiopulmonary exercise testing score for predicting outcomes in patients with heart failure. Am Heart J 2008;156(6):1177–83.

63. Perl L, Kheifets M, Guido A, et al, MITRA-EF study *. Acute reduction in left ventricular function following transcatheter mitral edge-to-edge repair. J Am Heart Assoc 2023;12(13):e029735.

64. Godino C, Munafo A, Scotti A, et al. MitraClip in secondary mitral regurgitation as a bridge to heart

transplantation: 1-year outcomes from the International MitraBridge Registry. J Heart Lung Transplant 2020;39(12):1353–62.

65. Giustino G, Lindenfeld J, Abraham WT, et al. NYHA functional classification and outcomes after transcatheter mitral valve repair in heart failure: The COAPT trial. JACC Cardiovasc Interv 2020;13(20):2317–28.

66. Adamo M, Tomasoni D, Stolz L, et al. Impact of transcatheter edge-to-edge mitral valve repair on guideline-directed medical therapy uptitration. JACC Cardiovasc Interv 2023;16(8):896–905.

67. Brener MI, Grayburn P, Lindenfeld J, et al. Right ventricular-pulmonary arterial coupling in patients with hf secondary MR: analysis from the COAPT trial. JACC Cardiovasc Interv 2021;14(20):2231–42.

68. Ben-Yehuda O, Shahim B, Chen S, et al. Pulmonary hypertension in transcatheter mitral valve repair for secondary mitral regurgitation: The COAPT trial. J Am Coll Cardiol 2020;76(22):2595–606.

69. Osteresch R, Diehl K, Kuhl M, et al. Impact of right heart function on outcome in patients with functional mitral regurgitation and chronic heart failure undergoing percutaneous edge-to-edge-repair. J Interv Cardiol 2018;31(6):916–24.

70. Ben-Shoshan J, Overtchook P, Buithieu J, et al. Predictors of outcomes following transcatheter edge-to-edge mitral valve repair. JACC Cardiovasc Interv 2020;13(15):1733–48.

71. Hahn RT, Asch F, Weissman NJ, et al. Impact of tricuspid regurgitation on clinical outcomes: The COAPT trial. J Am Coll Cardiol 2020;76(11):1305–14.

72. Cavalcante JL, Kusunose K, Obuchowski NA, et al. Prognostic impact of ischemic mitral regurgitation severity and myocardial infarct quantification by cardiovascular magnetic resonance. JACC Cardiovasc Imaging 2020;13(7):1489–501.

73. Levy WC, Mozaffarian D, Linker DT, et al. The seattle heart failure model: prediction of survival in heart failure. Circulation 2006;113(11):1424–33.

74. Morris AA, Khazanie P, Drazner MH, et al, American Heart Association Heart Failure and Transplantation Committee of the Council on Clinical Cardiology; Council on Arteriosclerosis, Thrombosis and Vascular Biology; Council on Cardiovascular Radiology and Intervention; and Council on Hypertension. Guidance for timely and appropriate referral of patients with advanced heart failure: a scientific statement from the american heart association. Circulation 2021;144(15):e238–50.

75. Koell B, Orban M, Weimann J, et al, EuroSMR Investigators. Outcomes stratified by adapted inclusion criteria after mitral edge-to-edge repair. J Am Coll Cardiol 2021;78(24):2408–21.

76. Grayburn PA, Sannino A, Packer M. Proportionate and disproportionate functional mitral regurgitation: a new conceptual framework that reconciles the results of the MITRA-FR and COAPT trials. JACC Cardiovasc Imaging 2019;12(2):353–62.

77. Claeys MJ, Debonnaire P, Bracke V, et al. Clinical and hemodynamic effects of percutaneous edge-to-edge mitral valve repair in atrial versus ventricular functional mitral regurgitation. Am J Cardiol 2021;161:70–5.

78. von Bardeleben RS, Mahoney P, Morse MA, et al. 1-Year Outcomes With Fourth-Generation Mitral Valve Transcatheter Edge-to-Edge Repair From the EXPAND G4 Study. J Am Coll Cardiol Intv 2023;16(21):2600–10.

79. Shuvy M, von Bardeleben RS, Grasso C, et al, EXPAND Investigators. Safety and efficacy of MitraClip in acutely ill (NYHA Class IV) patients with mitral regurgitation: Results from the global EXPAND study. ESC Heart Fail 2023;10(2):1122–32.

80. McDonagh TA, Metra M, Adamo M, et al, ESC Scientific Document Group. 2021 ESC Guidelines for the diagnosis and treatment of acute and chronic heart failure. Eur Heart J 2021;42(36):3599–726.

81. Simard T, Vemulapalli S, Jung RG, et al. Transcatheter edge-to-edge mitral valve repair in patients with severe mitral regurgitation and cardiogenic shock. J Am Coll Cardiol 2022;80(22):2072–84.

82. Parlow S, Di Santo P, Jung RG, et al. Transcatheter mitral valve repair for inotrope dependent cardiogenic shock - Design and rationale of the CAPITAL MINOS trial. Am Heart J 2022;254:81–7.

83. Sorajja P, Sato H, Bapat VN, et al. Contemporary anatomic criteria and clinical outcomes with transcatheter mitral repair. Circ Cardiovasc Interv 2023;16(2):e012486.

Functional Mitral Regurgitation
Transcatheter Therapy

Anita W. Asgar, MD, MSc

KEYWORDS

• Mitral regurgitation • Transcatheter therapy • Transcatheter edge-to-edge repair • Annuloplasty

KEY POINTS

- MR is separated into primary and secondary, differentiated by the presence of absence of pathology of the mitral valve or valvular apparatus.
- Secondary atrial MR or atrial functional MR typically occurs in the setting of atrial fibrillation and preserved left ventricular function.
- Secondary ventricular MR is very common, with an estimated prevalence of up to 50% in patients with ischemic or dilated cardiomyopathy.

INTRODUCTION

Mitral regurgitation (MR) is one of the most prevalent types of valvular heart disease and is expected to increase in the next decade.[1,2] Transcatheter therapies for MR are constantly being developed and studied for use in this population. In this review, the author describes the phenotypes of functional or secondary mitral regurgitation, discusses the potential therapeutic targets for transcatheter intervention, and reviews the results of such technology in the literature.

THE MITRAL VALVE AND PATHOPHYSIOLOGY OF SECONDARY MITRAL REGURGITATION

The mitral valve is a complex structure composed of the mitral valve annulus, valve leaflets, the supporting chordae tendinae, and the papillary muscles which insert directly into the wall of the left ventricle (LV). In addition, the left atrium is now recognized to play an important role in the development of mitral regurgitation (Fig. 1).

MR is separated into primary and secondary, differentiated by the presence of absence of pathology of the mitral valve or valvular apparatus. Secondary or functional mitral regurgitation, as it is often referred to, occurs in the setting of normal valve leaflets and subvalvular apparatus. It is now recognized to consist of two separate entities with distinct phenotypes: secondary atrial and secondary ventricular MR (Fig. 2).

Secondary atrial MR or atrial functional MR typically occurs in the setting of atrial fibrillation (AF) and preserved left ventricular function. The exact prevalence of this entity is unknown; however, estimates range from 7% in a population of patients with lone AF to up to 50% in those with heart failure preserved ejection fraction. The pathophysiology is felt to be dilatation of the left atrium in response to AF and subsequent dilation of the mitral annulus resulting in a lack of mitral leaflet coaptation and mitral regurgitation. The ventricle is typically not dilated; however, patients may have coexistent heart failure with preserved ejection fraction (HFpEF). Atrial functional MR may also occur in the absence of AF in patients with HFpEF with dilated left atria and concomitant mitral annular dilatation due to diastolic dysfunction and elevated left atrial pressures. Typical echocardiographic findings

Structural Heart Program, Montreal Heart Institute, 5000 rue Belanger, Montreal, H1T1C8 Canada
E-mail address: anita.asgar@gmail.com

Intervent Cardiol Clin 13 (2024) 183–189
https://doi.org/10.1016/j.iccl.2023.12.001
2211-7458/24/© 2023 Elsevier Inc. All rights reserved.

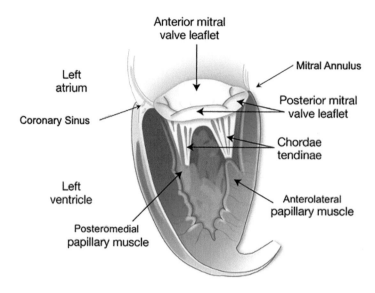

Fig. 1. Anatomy of the mitral valve.

Anterior mitral valve leaflet

Left atrium

Coronary Sinus

Left ventricle

Posteromedial papillary muscle

Mitral Annulus

Posterior mitral valve leaflet

Chordae tendinae

Anterolateral papillary muscle

include an enlarged left atrium, normal left ventricular systolic function, normal leaflet motion, but a central regurgitant jet with leaflet coaptation occurring at the annular level and a lack of coaptation reserve.[3]

Secondary ventricular MR is very common, with an estimated prevalence of up to 50% in patients with ischemic or dilated cardiomyopathy. This phenotype is characterized by LV dilation due to ischemic or nonischemic cardiomyopathy which secondarily impairs leaflet coaptation of a structurally normal MV. Specifically, LV dysfunction and remodeling lead to apical and lateral papillary muscle displacement, which results in leaflet tethering, dilation, and flattening of the mitral annulus, and therefore reduced closing forces of the mitral valve.

Ventricular secondary MR can be classified as either ischemic or nonischemic. In ischemic MR due to previous myocardial infarction, LV remodeling results in papillary muscle displacement, causing systolic tenting of the mitral valve even in the absence of a significant reduction in left ventricular ejection fraction (LVEF). In fact, regional wall motion abnormalities with remodeling may result in sufficient MV tethering to cause severe MR, despite preserved LV function. Nonischemic MR, most commonly due to hypertension or dilated cardiomyopathy, is categorized by global LV dilation with increased sphericity and (typically) a centrally located regurgitant jet. Symmetric mitral annular dilation is greatest in the septal-lateral direction and correlates with the severity of LV dysfunction.[4]

THERAPEUTIC TARGETS FOR THE TREATMENT OF SECONDARY MITRAL REGURGITATION

Treatment for secondary MR is based on a pyramidal approach built on a foundation of guideline-directed medical therapy for heart failure with reduced or preserved ejection fraction (Fig. 3). Patients with reduced ejection fraction require optimization with the four classes of medical therapy including beta-blockers, mineralocorticoid receptor antagonists, sacubitril/valsartan and the newest class sodium glucose co-transporter 2 inhibitors (SGLT2is), and cardiac resynchronization therapy as indicated. In the setting of HFpEF, medical therapy consists of use of SGLT2i (Class of Recommendation 2a), mineralocorticoid receptor antagonist (MRAs) (Class of Recommendation 2b), and angiotensin receptor/neprilysin inhibitor (ARNi) (Class of Recommendation 2b).[5] Persistent secondary MR despite medical therapy may be addressable using transcatheter therapies targeting various parts of the mitral valve.

Transcatheter therapies for functional mitral regurgitation have been designed to address different anatomic aspects of the mitral valve, as shown in Table 1. Specifically, devices have targeted mitral annular reduction via direct or indirect approaches to perform mitral annuloplasty. Such devices include the Cardioband (Edwards LIfeSciences, Irvine, CA) for direct annuloplasty, using a device that is delivered via transseptal puncture and anchors directly into the mitral annulus, and the Carillon device (Cardiac Dimensions) for indirect annuloplasty using implantation in the

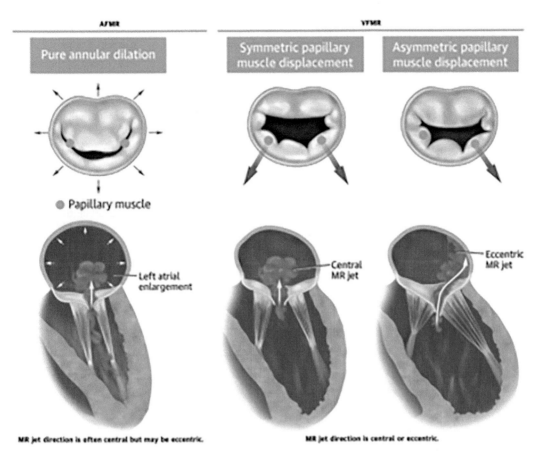

Fig. 2. Phenotypes of secondary mitral regurgitation: atrial and ventricular.

coronary sinus. The mitral valve leaflets have been primarily addressed using leaflet approximation or transcatheter edge-to-edge repair (TEER) using the MitraClip device (Abbott, Menlo Park, CA) in functional mitral regurgitation (FMR). An additional device for TEER, PASCAL (Edwards LifeSciences, Irvine, CA) is now approved for degenerative or primary MR with results awaited from the trial in functional MR. Alternative approaches include basal ventricular wall cinching to create left ventricular remodeling at the basal ventricular level using a

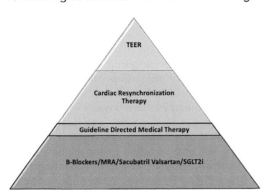

Fig. 3. Pyramidal approach to the treatment of secondary MR.

device called Accucinch (Ancora Heart). This device was initially designed to target FMR but is now refocussing on cardiac remodeling for heart failure and is described as a ventricular restoration therapy that is being studied in the CORCINCH-HF trial (NCT04331769), therefore will not be discussed further in this review.

Most of these devices are in the research stages however current guideline recommendations support the use of TEER or TEER with the MitraClip device (2a recommendation) in patients meeting inclusion criteria for the COAPT (Cardiovascular Outcomes Assessment of the MitraClip Percutaneous Therapy for Heart Failure Patients with Functional Mitral Regurgitation) trial, specifically severe secondary MR with suitable anatomy for TEER: LVEF 20% to 50%, LVESD ≤70 mm, and PASP ≤70 mm Hg.[6]

DATA ON TRANSCATHETER THERAPIES FOR SECONDARY MITRAL REGURGITATION
Transcatheter Edge-to-Edge Repair
The most studied device for secondary MR is the MitraClip for edge-to-edge repair, with two

Table 1
Transcatheter therapies for the treatment of functional mitral regurgitation

Device	Anatomic Target	Mechanism of Action	Current Status
MitraClip	Valve leaflets	Leaflet approximation and restoration of leaflet coaptation	*FDA approval* for the treatment of secondary MR, high-risk primary MR (US) *CE mark* in Europe
Pascal	Valve leaflets	Leaflet approximation and restoration of leaflet coaptation	Currently enrolling in the CLASP IIF trial in secondary MR *FDA approval* in high-risk primary MR (US) *CE mark* in Europe
Cardioband	Mitral annulus	Annular reduction via direct traction on the posterior mitral annulus	*CE mark* in Europe
Carillon	Coronary sinus	Annular reduction via pressure on the posterior annulus from the coronary sinus	*CE mark* in Europe

randomized controlled trials (RCTs) in secondary MR: COAPT and the MITRA-FR (Percutaneous Repair with the MitraClip Device for Severe Functional/Secondary Mitral Regurgitation) trial.

The COAPT trial randomized 614 patients in 78 centers in the United States and Canada, with symptomatic moderate to severe or severe secondary MR despite maximal guideline-directed medical treatment for heart failure to continued medical therapy or the MitraClip device in a 1:1 ratio.[7] The primary effectiveness endpoint was all heart failure-related hospitalizations within 24 months and the primary safety endpoint was freedom from device-related complications at 12 months. Important secondary endpoints included all-cause mortality, quality of life, functional capacity, MR reduction, and left ventricular remodeling. At 24 months, rate of all hospitalizations for heart failure was 35.8% per patient-year in the device group as compared with 67.9% per patient-year in the control group (hazard ratio (HR) 0.53; 95% confidence interval [CI], 0.40–0.70; $P < .001$) with a number needed to treat of 3.1 patients. The safety endpoint of freedom from device-related complications at 12 months was 96.6% (lower 95% confidence limit, 94.8%; $P < .001$ for comparison with the performance goal). Secondary endpoints of death from any cause within 24 months occurred in 29.1% of the patients in the device group as compared with 46.1% in the control group (HR 0.62; 95% CI, 0.46–0.82; $P < .001$). The number needed to treat to save one life by 24 months was 5.9 (95% CI, 3.9–11.7). The positivity of this trial lead to FDA approval of the device for the treatment of secondary MR and inclusion in the guidelines for the treatment of heart failure and secondary MR.[6]

The MITRA-FR trial was a trial of 307 patients performed in 37 centers in France of patients with severe secondary mitral regurgitation and symptomatic heart failure, randomized in a 1:1 ratio to medical therapy or treatment with Mitra-Clip. The primary efficacy outcome was a composite of death from any cause or unplanned hospitalization for heart failure at 12 months after randomization. Secondary outcomes included death from cardiac causes, survival from major adverse cardiovascular events including stroke at 12 months and echocardiographic endpoints including MR reduction and left ventricular remodeling. At 12 months, there was no difference between medical therapy and MitraClip for the primary composite endpoint.[8] Extended follow-up to 24 months also failed to show a difference between the two cohorts with the composite of all-cause death and unplanned hospitalization for heart failure occurring in 63.8% of patients (97/152) in the intervention group and 67.1% (102/152) in the control group (HR 1.01, 95% CI 0.77 to 1.34). The individual component of all-cause mortality occurred in 34.9% of patients (53/152) in the intervention group and 34.2% (52/152) in the control group (HR 1.02, 95% CI 0.70–1.50) and unplanned hospitalization for heart failure occurred in 55.9% of patients (85/152) in the intervention group and 61.8% (94/152) in the control group (HR 0.97, 95% CI 0.72–1.30).[9]

The follow-up of the COAPT trial was recently presented and published and provided a longer term perspective on the outcomes of these patients. At 5 years, there continued to be a statistically significant difference in heart failure hospitalizations between MitraClip therapy and medical therapy, 33.1% per year in the device group and 57.2% per year in the control group (HR 0.53; 95% CI, 0.41–0.68). In addition, all-cause mortality was 57.3% in the device group and 67.2% in the control group (HR 0.72; 95% CI, 0.58–0.89). Death or hospitalization for heart failure within 5 years occurred in 73.6% of the patients in the device group and in 91.5% of those in the control group (HR, 0.53; 95% CI, 0.44–0.64) highlighting the overall high risk of this patient population and the prognosis of the disease.[10] Interestingly, the patients in the medical treatment arm that crossed over to MitraClip after 2 years seemed to have similar benefit in terms of HF hospitalizations and mortality as those initially treated with MitraClip.

There has been much debate about the differing outcomes in these two trials, which on the surface seem very similar. There are however important differences that may or may not have led to the differing outcomes. First, the severity of MR in the two trials were not the same due to the different definitions of MR severity,

specifically the utilization of a lower threshold of effective regurgitant orifice and regurgitant volume in the MITRA-FR trials, resulting in what would be defined as more moderate MR according to the American Society of Echo Guidelines.[11] Second, medical therapy was not closely monitored or up-titrated in MITRA-FR as compared with the rather stringent protocol used in COAPT. There have been numerous other theories proposed for the differing outcomes and 5 years later, the debate remains unresolved.

What has become clear is the complexity and nuance associated with the management of secondary MR patients in the landscape of evolving medical therapy and device improvements and iterations. In fact, the disease itself is likely a spectrum of severity in which patient benefit from TEER may depend most on the stage at which intervention is performed. A recent analysis of the EuroSMR (European Registry of Transcatheter Repair for Secondary Mitral Regurgitation), a retrospective registry of mitral TEER patients undergoing treatment at 11 cardiac centers across Europe from 2008 to 2019 evaluated the concept of disease staging the relationship to patient outcomes. Disease stages were created based on echocardiographic and clinical evaluation and patients were assigned to one of the following four groups: left ventricular involvement (Stage 1), left atrial involvement (Stage 2), right ventricular volume/pressure overload (Stage 3), or biventricular failure (Stage 4). A total of 849 patients were assigned to the four groups, 9.5% (n = 81) with left ventricular involvement (Stage 1), 46% (n = 393) with left atrial involvement (Stage 2), 15% (n = 129) with right ventricular pressure/volume overload (Stage 3), and 29% (n = 246) with biventricular failure (Stage 4). An increase in stage was associated with increased 2-year all-cause mortality after M-TEER (HR: 1.39; CI: 1.23–1.58; $P < .01$), and higher stages were associated with significantly less improvement in NYHA class at follow-up.[12]

As previously mentioned, secondary atrial MR is also an important phenotype of patients with secondary MR. Although there has yet to be randomized data in this specific group, registry data have demonstrated clinical benefit of TEER in this patient population. The EuroSMR registry has published data on this population as well. In the overall registry cohort of 1608 patients, 7.8% (n = 126) were identified as having secondary atrial MR. TEER was successful in this group with procedural success of 87.2% ($P<.001$) and significant improvement in the New York Heart

Association (NYHA) functional class (NYHA functional class III/IV: 86.5% at baseline to 36.6% at follow-up; $P<.001$). The estimated 2-year survival rate in secondary atrial MR patients was 70.4%. Two-year survival did not differ significantly between secondary atrial MR, non-atrial MR, and secondary ventricular MR. The predictors of 2-year survival in the atrial secondary MR group included advanced HF symptoms (baseline NYHA functional class IV), and right ventricular dysfunction (HR: 2.82 [95% CI: 1.24–6.45]; $P=.014$).[13]

Transcatheter Direct Mitral Annuloplasty

Transcatheter annular reduction has been studied using the Cardioband device in a single-arm multicenter prospective trial of patients with secondary MR. Inclusion criteria included age greater than 18 years, symptomatic patients with at least moderate or severe secondary MR and high surgical risk as assessed by the local heart team. Patients were treated with the Cardioband procedure, and technical, device, and procedural success were evaluated using the Mitral Valve Academic Research Consortium criteria. The results were as follows: technical success 97% (58/60), device success 72% (43/60), and procedural success 68% (41/60). At 12 months, overall survival, survival free of readmission for heart failure, and survival free of reintervention (performed in seven patients) were 87%, 66%, and 78%, respectively. There was evidence of reduction in mitral regurgitation; MR grade at 12 months was moderate or less in 61% of the overall cohort. There was also evidence of improvement in functional status and quality of life as assessed by the Minnesota Living with Heart Failure Questionnaire.[14]

The device is currently in RCTs and has Conformite Europeenne (CE) mark in Europe.

Transcatheter Indirect Mitral Annuloplasty

Annular reduction via an indirect approach using the Carillon device uses the anatomic relationship of the coronary sinus to the posterior mitral annulus to remodel the mitral annulus. The device has been studied in secondary MR in the REDUCE FMR trial.[15] This blinded, randomized, sham-controlled trial studied 120 patients receiving optimal heart failure medical therapy that were assigned to a coronary sinus-based mitral annular reduction approach for secondary MR or sham procedure. The primary endpoint was change in mitral regurgitant volume at 12 months, measured by echocardiography. The device was successfully implanted in 84% of study subjects. At 12 months, there was a statistically significant reduction in mitral regurgitant volume in the treatment group compared with the control group. In addition, there was a significant reduction in left ventricular volumes in patients receiving the device versus those in the control arm. It is important to note that 25% of patients in the control arm and 39% of patients in the treatment arm have only moderate mitral regurgitation. Clinical endpoints such as hospitalizations for heart failure or mortality were not evaluated as part of the primary endpoints.

A subsequent publication addressed the secondary endpoints of change from baseline in six minute walk test (6MWT) distance, NYHA class, and Kansas City Cardiomyopathy Questionnaire (KCCQ) as well as the incidence of HF hospitalization or death through 1 year of follow-up. The investigators defined the minimum clinically important difference (MCID) as a ≥ 30 m increase in 6MWT distance, an NYHA decrease in ≥ 1 class, and a ≥ 3 point increase in KCCQ score. At 1 year, the outcomes achieving an MCID were numerically higher in those treated with the Carillon device although not statistically significant, including freedom from heart failure hospitalization or death.[16]

Both devices have approval in Europe; however, clinical uptake is somewhat limited due to a lack of large randomized clinical trials and reimbursement challenges.

SUMMARY

Secondary MR is prevalent in the heart failure population, and there are multiple transcatheter therapies to address this problem. All therapy should be considered as additional to a foundation of guideline-directed medical therapy. Current transcatheter approaches target specific anatomic structures to reduce mitral regurgitation severity. At present, edge-to-edge repair has the most clinical data and is approved in both Europe and the United States to treat such patients.

CLINICS CARE POINTS

- Secondary mitral regurgitation (MR) has two distinct phenotypes: atrial functional MR and ventricular functional MR. Treatment of MR is based on a foundation of guideline-directed medical therapy for the underlying condition.

- Current transcatheter approaches to the treatment of secondary MR target the individual anatomic components of the mitral valve. Most devices remain in the investigational phase with only transcatheter edge-to-edge repair with the MitraClip approved in North America for the treatment of secondary MR.

- Randomized controlled trial data have demonstrated improvements in heart failure hospitalizations and all-cause mortality in secondary MR treated with the MitraClip device.
- Transcatheter therapy of secondary MR may be considered in patients as part of a pyramidal approach to the treatment of heart failure and secondary MR. The current guidelines support use of the only approved device, MitraClip as a 2A recommendation (American College of Cardiology/ American Heart Association [ACC/AHA] guidelines), and the European guidelines.

DISCLOSURE

Consultant/research support Abbott, Edwards LifeSciences.

REFERENCES

1. Nkomo VT, Gardin JM, Gottdiener JS, et al. Burden of valvular heart diseases: a population- based study. Lancet 2006;368:1005–11.
2. De Marchena E, Badiye A, Robalino G, et al. Respective prevalence of the different Carpentier classes of mitral regurgitation: a stepping stone for future therapeutic research and development. J Card Surg 2011;26:385–92.
3. Deferm S, Bertrand PB, Verbrugge FH, et al. Atrial functional mitral regurgitation: JACC review topic of the week. J Am Coll Cardiol 2019;73(19):2465–76.
4. Asgar AW, Mack MJ, Stone GW. Secondary mitral regurgitation in heart failure: pathophysiology, prognosis, and therapeutic considerations. J Am Coll Cardiol 2015;65(12):1231–48. Erratum in: J Am Coll Cardiol. 2015 May 26;65(20):2265. PMID: 25814231.
5. Heidenreich PA, Bozkurt B, Aguilar D, et al. 2022 AHA/ACC/HFSA guideline for the management of heart failure: a report of the American college of cardiology/American heart association joint committee on clinical practice guidelines. Circulation 2022;145(18): e895–1032. Epub 2022 Apr 1. Erratum in: Circulation. 2022 May 3;145(18):e1033. Erratum in: Circulation. 2022 Sep 27;146(13):e185. Erratum in: Circulation. 2023 Apr 4;147(14):e674. PMID: 35363499.
6. Otto CM, Nishimura RA, Bonow RO, et al. 2020 ACC/AHA Guideline for the Management of Patients With Valvular Heart Disease: Executive Summary: A Report of the American College of Cardiology/American Heart Association Joint Committee on Clinical Practice Guidelines. Circulation 2021;143(5):e35–71. Erratum in: Circulation. 2021 Feb 2;143(5):e228. Erratum in: Circulation. 2021 Mar 9;143(10):e784. PMID: 33332149.
7. Stone GW, Lindenfeld J, Abraham WT, et al, COAPT Investigators. Transcatheter mitral-valve repair in patients with heart failure. N Engl J Med 2018;379:2307–18.
8. Obadia J-F, Messika-Zeitoun D, Leurent G, et al, MITRA-FR Investigators. Percutaneous repair or medical treatment for secondary mitral regurgitation. N Engl J Med 2018;379:2297–306.
9. Iung B, Armoiry X, Vahanian A, et al. Percutaneous repair or medical treatment for secondary mitral regurgitation: outcomes at 2 years. Eur J Heart Fail 2019;21(12):1619–27.
10. Stone GW, Abraham WT, Lindenfeld J, et al, COAPT Investigators. Five-year follow-up after transcatheter repair of secondary mitral regurgitation. N Engl J Med 2023;388:2037–48.
11. Zoghbi WA, Adams D, Bonow RO, et al. Recommendations for noninvasive evaluation of native valvular regurgitation: a report from the American society of echocardiography developed in collaboration with the society for cardiovascular magnetic resonance. J Am Soc Echocardiogr 2017;30(4): 303–71.
12. Stolz L, Doldi PM, Orban M, et al. Staging heart failure patients with secondary mitral regurgitation undergoing transcatheter edge-to-edge repair. JACC Cardiovasc Interv 2023;16(2): 140–51.
13. Doldi P, Stolz L, Orban M, et al. Transcatheter mitral valve repair in patients with atrial functional mitral regurgitation. JACC Cardiovasc Imaging 2022;15(11):1843–51.
14. Messika-Zeitoun D, Nickenig G, Latib A, et al. Transcatheter mitral valve repair for functional mitral regurgitation using the Cardioband system: 1 year outcomes. Eur Heart J 2019 Feb 1;40(5):466–72.
15. Witte KK, Lipiecki J, Siminiak T, et al. The REDUCE FMR trial: a randomized sham-controlled study of percutaneous mitral annuloplasty in functional mitral regurgitation. JACC Heart Fail 2019 Nov; 7(11):945–55.
16. Khan MS, Siddiqi TJ, Butler J, et al. Functional outcomes with Carillon device over 1 year in patients with functional mitral regurgitation of Grades 2+ to 4+: results from the REDUCE-FMR trial. ESC Heart Fail 2021 Apr; 8(2):872–8.

Mitral Regurgitation Complicated by Cardiogenic Shock

Reassessing Risk Stratification and Therapeutic Strategies

Carla Boyle, BSc, Khoa Nguyen, MD,
Johannes Steiner, MD, Conrad J. Macon, MD,
Jeffrey A. Marbach, MBBS, MS*

KEYWORDS

- Cardiogenic shock • Mitral regurgitation • Risk stratification • Therapeutic strategies

---

KEY POINTS

- The management of acute mitral regurgitation (MR) complicated by cardiogenic shock (CS) is a complex and challenging task.
- Early identification and risk stratification of patients with acute MR and CS is crucial, and the integration of invasive hemodynamic monitoring is essential in guiding therapeutic strategies.
- Temporary mechanical circulatory support devices, such as intra-aortic balloon pump (IABP) and Impella-CP, offer valuable options in stabilizing patients and bridging them to definitive management.
- Transcatheter edge-to-edge repair with devices like MitraClip and PASCAL provide promising alternatives for patients at high surgical risk.

INTRODUCTION

Cardiogenic shock (CS) is a severe manifestation of acute decompensated heart failure characterized by insufficient cardiac output (CO), leading to tissue hypoperfusion and eventual end-organ failure.[1–3] Mitral regurgitation (MR) is the most common valvular disorder in the world, occurring in up to 2% of the world's population.[4] While two distinct cardiovascular pathologies, CS and MR frequently coexist, and the complex interplay between them significantly alters risk stratification and the therapeutic strategies available to patients.[5,6]

From a clinical viewpoint, MR can be broadly categorized into either primary or secondary.[7]

Primary MR is the result of an intrinsic (organic or degenerative) valvular process, such as a spontaneous chordal rupture or leaflet perforation. Secondary or functional MR is the consequence of disease of the left ventricle and/or mitral valve annulus.[5,8] Though primary and secondary MR are two discrete pathologies, there is frequent overlap between the two.

MR can be further classified according to its chronicity. Chronic MR develops over many years and is often well compensated due to left ventricular dilation enabling maintenance of forward stroke volume. Acute MR, on the other hand, generates a rapid and severe rise in both left atrial volume and pressure as a direct consequence of the newly incompetent mitral

---

Division of Cardiology, Knight Cardiovascular Institute, Oregon Health & Science University, 3161 Southwest Pavilion Loop, Portland, OR 97239, USA

* Corresponding author. Interventional Cardiology & Cardiac Critical Care, Knight Cardiovascular Institute, Oregon Health & Science University, UHN-62, 3161, Southwest Pavilion Loop, Portland, OR 97239.
E-mail address: marbach@ohsu.edu

Intervent Cardiol Clin 13 (2024) 191–205
https://doi.org/10.1016/j.iccl.2023.11.003

valve.[5,7,8] The clinical result of this abrupt hemo-dynamic change is acute pulmonary edema and a reduced forward stroke volume, the combina-tion of which may precipitate acute CS and re-quires urgent treatment.[9] Distinguishing between these two distinctly different entities is crucial in understanding hemodynamic alter-ations, risk stratifying patients, and predicting response to treatment.

In this review, we will focus our attention on the immediate and definitive management strate-gies available to patients with acute MR compli-cated by CS, including the hemodynamic and prognostic indicators utilized in assessing CS severity. By integrating current evidence and clin-ical guidelines, the authors outline the ideal ther-apeutic approaches and highlight emerging technologies that hold promise in improving out-comes for this complex population.

RISK STRATIFICATION & INITIAL MANAGEMENT

Definitive therapy in patients with acute MR generally require a mechanical solution, which may be surgical or transcatheter based. Howev-er, definitive therapies take time to plan and require some degree of hemodynamic stability. Therefore, swift interventions to stabilize the he-modynamic perturbations and prevent the onset of multi-organ dysfunction are critical in the setting of acute MR.

Although data specific to patients with acute MR complicated by CS are limited, the authors advocate for initial risk stratification in this pop-ulation to mirror the Society of Cardiovascular Angiography and Intervention (SCAI) shock stage classification system.[10,11] Specific princi-ples that are felt to be fundamental to the early evaluation and management of patients with acute MR are (1) urgent identification and evalu-ation of patients with overt or suspected CS, (2) early hemodynamic profiling and initiation of vasoactive and/or temporary mechanical cir-culatory support (t-MCS), and (3) continuous he-modynamic monitoring to direct escalation or de-escalation of therapies.[12–14] For the majority of patients with acute MR, this requires manage-ment in a critical care setting where invasive he-modynamics can be monitored, and vasoactive medications can be administered.

While the use of pulmonary artery catheters (PAC) for hemodynamic assessment and moni-toring in patients with CS declined by approxi-mately 75% between 2000 and 2014, recent data has suggested that complete invasive he-modynamic profiling is fundamental for diag-nosing, risk stratifying, and guiding therapy among all-comer CS cohorts.[15–18] This allows for phenotyping of the degree of hemodynamic compromise as well as monitoring of the response to therapies with parameters such as pulmonary capillary wedge pressure (PCWP) and systemic cardiac output (CO)/cardiac index (CI). Fig. 1 outlines a general approach to pa-tient phenotyping and escalation of support in the setting of hemodynamic deterioration, with the ultimate goal of stabilizing the patient (Stage A-B) so that they may undergo definitive therapy.[19]

Afterload Reduction

Vasopressors and inotropes are the most frequently utilized strategy for providing hemo-dynamic support in patients with CS. However, increasing vasopressor and inotropic support has been demonstrated to increase myocardial oxygen demand at a time of reduced coronary blood flow, thereby exacerbating the supply-demand imbalance, and resulting in detrimental

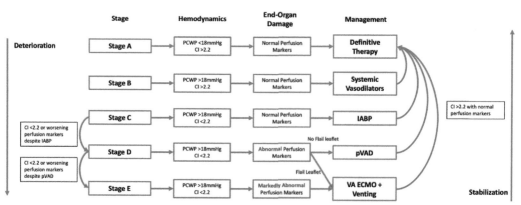

Fig. 1. Approach to management of mitral regurgitation complicated by cardiogenic shock. Stages are based on Society of Cardiovascular Angiography and Intervention (SCAI) shock stages.

effects on myocyte function.[12,20] Moreover, vasopressors induce systemic vasoconstriction and may exacerbate peripheral organ hypoperfusion.[21] These hemodynamic effects may be particularly harmful in patients with acute MR, where an increase in afterload and CO may serve only to increase the regurgitant fraction, as opposed to the forward stroke volume.

Initial medical management, therefore, should be targeted at afterload reduction with systemic vasodilators, with the goal of maximizing forward stroke volume and minimizing the regurgitant fraction in attempt to maintain adequate tissue perfusion.[11,22–24] The preferred systemic vasodilator for acute MR is nitroprusside, which upon being metabolized to nitric oxide results in potent arterial and venous vasodilation, providing both a reduction in systemic vascular resistance and an increase in venous capacitance.[25] Together, these effects manifest as a decrease in PCWP, a decrease mean arterial pressure (MAP), a reduction in regurgitant fraction, and an increase in CO, all while having a neutral effect on cardiac contractility and inotropy.[24,26–28] Evidence of these beneficial effects has been observed in several clinical scenarios. In one cohort of patients with severe low-output heart failure, a retrospective analysis found that patients who were treated with nitroprusside (N = 78) achieved a greater reduction in intracardiac filling pressures compared to those treated with inotropes (N = 97).[25] Similarly, among patients with severe MR (N = 8) treatment with nitroprusside led to a significant decrease in left ventricle (LV) filling pressures (33 ± 1.8–16 ± 1.4 mm Hg), an increase in forward CI (2.2 ± 3.5–3.3 ± 0.47 L/min/M^2) and forward stroke volume index (23 ± 4.4–36 ± 6.6 mL/M^2) along with a reduction in systemic vascular resistance (1802 ± 331–1102 ± 241 dyn/sec/cm^{-5}).[26] Finally, the extremely short half-life (approximately 2 minutes) allows rapid titration according to hemodynamic requirements and makes it an ideal therapy in the setting of severe MR and CS.[29]

Another class of systemic vasodilators that are potentially beneficial in this clinical scenario is the dihydropyridine calcium channel blockers (ie, nicardipine, clevidipine). While they also possess rapid acting pharmacologic effects, they lack the venodilatory effects of nitroprusside. Additionally, the negative inotropic properties of nicardipine are of theoretic concern, though the clinical significance of this is questionable.[30] Clevidipine is felt to be more selective and has less negative inotropic effects.[31]

Intra-aortic Balloon Pump

Despite vasodilators possessing ideal pharmacologic properties for the treatment of acute MR, many patients will be unable to tolerate vasodilators or will fail to adequately respond. In one analysis of patients with acute MR in the setting of acute myocardial infarction complicated by CS (AMI-CS), escalation to t-MCS was required in over two-thirds of patients prior to definitive surgical management.[32] For those unable to tolerate vasodilators or who do not recover to a Stage B profile, t-MCS with an intra-aortic balloon pump (IABP) is the preferred escalation strategy for most patients.[33,34]

While routine treatment with an IABP was not found to improve outcomes among patients with AMI-CS, its value in the setting of acute MR complicated by CS may result from the hemodynamic differences between these two conditions.[35] In AMI-CS, the IABP provides approximately 0.5 L/min of CO through a reduction in left ventricular afterload in systole and increased mean coronary blood flow in diastole.[14,36] In acute MR, however, despite a marginal decrease in afterload due to competing retrograde impedance, the systolic deflation of the IABP shifts the ratio of regurgitant to antegrade flow, leading to a 31% increase in systemic CO, up to as much as a 1 L/min.[37] These hemodynamic benefits, combined with the more favorable side effect profile, compared to alternative t-MCS devices, make the IABP an ideal first choice for those with acute MR as a bridge to definitive therapies. Though large randomized clinical trials to support this recommendation are lacking, retrospective data have demonstrated a reduction in 30-day mortality among patients with acute MR, primarily driven by a reduction in preoperative mortality.[38]

Axial Flow Pumps

For individuals exhibiting indications of end-organ impairment or those still unable to sustain adequate forward blood flow (cardiac index < 2.0 L/min/m^2) despite vasodilators and/or IABP, a more robust mechanical support strategy becomes imperative. The primary device employed under these circumstances is the Impella-CP (Abiomed, Danvers, Massachusetts). This t-MCS device is a percutaneous, micro-axial flow pump that propels blood from the left ventricle into the ascending aorta using an Archimedes screw design, and is able to generate continuous flow up to 3.5 to 4.0 L/min.[39]

The feasibility of this device as a bridge to definitive management in patients with acute MR complicated by CS was demonstrated in a small cohort study, where 86% of patients who were managed with an Impella CP prior to MitraClip (Abbott Vascular, Abbott Park, Illinois) survived to hospital discharge.[40] In contrast to the IABP, the Impella CP device provides superior hemodynamic support but carries a greater risk due to a larger bore femoral sheath (14 Fr), potential for hemolysis, the necessity for frequent repositioning, and systemic anticoagulation to mitigate the risk of thrombus formation along the catheter or device body. Furthermore, in the setting of a flail mitral valve leaflet, placement of the Impella devices may not be feasible given concerns for entanglement of the flailed leaflet with the device motor leading to further leaflet destruction. This, however, is a theoretic concern with several case reports and case series demonstrating instances in which the use of an intraventricular Impella has been safely accomplished.[41,42]

An alternative t-MCS device is the Tandem-Heart (LivaNova, London, UK), an extracorporeal system in which the drainage canula is percutaneously placed through the femoral vein and into the left atrium via a transeptal puncture, and the arterial return cannula is placed in the femoral artery. In cases of refractory hypoxemia from acute pulmonary edema, an oxygenator can be spliced into the circuit akin to peripheral veno-arterial extracorporeal membrane oxygenation (VA-ECMO). As it is not an intraventricular device, the theoretic concerns of a flail leaflet are absent. In at least one case series, this arrangement has proven to be a viable choice for guiding patients toward surgery and recovery.[43] However, challenges such as the expertise needed to position the device across the atrial septum and its instability in this placement highlight potential drawbacks.

Veno-Arterial Extracorporeal Membrane Oxygenation
Individuals who do not respond to or who are rapidly deteriorating despite vasodilators and/or t-MCS devices may require immediate escalation to veno-arterial extracorporeal membrane oxygenation (VA-ECMO), though this is infrequent, being necessary in less than 5% of individuals with acute MR.[33] Compared to the aforementioned t-MCS devices, VA-ECMO offers increased hemodynamic support but also entails a higher complication rate. As a consequence, the survival rate for those with AMR on VA-ECMO is only 61.9%, which can largely be attributed to common complications such as limb ischemia (16.9%), amputation (4.7%), stroke (5.9%), kidney injury leading to dialysis (46%), and infection (30%).[44,45]

In most configurations of VA-ECMO, a 21 to 25 French drainage cannula in the femoral vein pulls blood from the right atrium leading to a decrease in the right atrial and pulmonary artery pressures. Deoxygenated blood is then pumped through an oxygenator and into the femoral artery through a 15 to 19 French return cannula. To prevent lower extremity ischemia distal to the arterial return cannula, a distal perfusion sheath is often used.[46,47] Although peripheral VA-ECMO greatly increases the blood flow to the rest of the body, it can have deleterious effects on the heart. The retrograde blood flow up the descending aorta from the arterial cannula increases the impedance to blood flow out of the left ventricle. This increased impedance to forward flow increases the regurgitant flow and can worsen MR. Thus, some type of "venting" strategy to mitigate this increased impediment to flow is necessary in VA-ECMO used in acute MR.

The most commonly employed strategy to "vent" the LV is through insertion of an Impella-CP to prevent deleterious effects on the LV while bridging toward definitive surgery.[48] When there is a flailed anterior mitral leaflet with anatomy not suitable for Impella device placement, alternative strategies include using an IABP, creating an atrial septostomy, or percutaneous placement of a drainage cannula in the left atrium (Table 1).[41,49]

DEFINITIVE MANAGEMENT
Surgical Mitral Valve Replacement and Transcatheter Edge-To-Edge Repair
Timely mitral valve (MV) repair or replacement can be a life-saving measure in the setting of CS secondary to or complicated by acute MR. According to the 2020 American College of Cardiology(ACC)/American Heart Association(AHA) valvular heart disease guidelines, surgical MV repair remains the preferred intervention in the setting of acute, primary MR.[5] In several clinical scenarios including papillary muscle rupture and infective endocarditis, surgical treatment—in fact—is the only viable option.[50] Unfortunately, postsurgical mortality in the setting of severe MR and CS remains extremely high and consequently, many patients are deemed to be at prohibitive risk for surgery.

Therapeutic options are even more limited in secondary MR associated with cardiogenic shock. Untreated secondary MR with CS is associated with an 80% mortality rate which is only reduced to approximately 53% with surgical intervention.[51] In recent years, percutaneous MV repair and replacement options have emerged and can

Table 1
Outcome data for mechanical circulatory support devices in mitral regurgitation

Authors Year	No. of Patients	Age (Mean)	Etiology	Intervention	Pre-Operative Mortality	Perioperative Mortality	Survival to Discharge	30-d Mortality	6-mo Mortality	Comments
Kettner et al.[38] 2013	20	64 ± 9	Acute MR c/b CS	IABP (Data scope Models 98, cs100 and cs 300)	IABP: 11% No IABP: 88%	IABP: 36%	-	61% (with IABP) 100% (No IABP)	-	This model of IABP was recalled in 2014 due to potential mechanical failure due to overheating
Jalil B et al.[39] 2017	1	59	Acute MR c/b CS	Impella 2.5	-	-	-	-	-	Use of Impella improved CO, pulmonary edema, hypoxia, vasopressor requirements and allowed MVR within 1 h of Impella placement.
Vandenbriele et al.[40] 2021	6	66.8 ± 4.9 y	Acute MR c/b CS	Impella CP & MitraClip	0%	-	86% (5/6)	-	86% (100% of discharged)	Non-survivor died of multi-organ failure that was present before intervention
DiVita et al.[43] 2020	2	48	Acute MR c/b CS	TandemHeart with Oxygenator	-	-	-	-	-	Two patient case studies. Both patients triaged as high surgical risk, and use of TandemHeart + Oxygenator stabilized hypoxia and

(continued on next page)

Table 1
(continued)

Authors Year	No. of Patients	Age (Mean)	Etiology	Intervention	Pre-Operative Mortality	Perioperative Mortality	Survival to Discharge	30-d Mortality	6-mo Mortality	Comments
										hemodynamic parameters to successfully bridge to surgery.
Ekanem et al.[48] 2020	3	65	Acute MR c/b CS	Impella CP & VA-ECMO	-	-	66%	-	-	Three patient case studies. Use of combined Impella-CV and VA ECMO stabilized patients to receive definitive surgical treatment. Non-survivor's hemodynamic values stabilized but later suffered a stroke and pneumonia leading to rapid deterioration.

Abbreviations: c/b, complicated by; CO, cardiac output; CS, cardiogenic shock; IABP, intra-aortic balloon pump; MR, mitral regurgitation; MVR, mitral valve replacement; VA-ECMO, veno-arterial extracorporeal membrane oxygenation.

offer alternative approaches for patients with appropriate anatomy at high or prohibitive surgical risk.[23]

Transcatheter edge-to-edge repairs (TEER) are increasingly being used as definitive treatments for MR in patients who are at high or prohibitive surgical risk. The MitraClip (Abbott Vascular, Abbott Park, Illinois) is perhaps the most established treatment, having been widely used since 2003. Outcomes with the MitraClip have been described in studies starting with the EVEREST series of trials focused in primary MR and most recently from the multicenter EXPAND and COAPT studies.[52,53] With the introduction of the next generation MitraClip NTR and XTR systems, approximately 87% of the patients have mild (1+) or less MR in post-market studies and registries compared with only 43% observed during the EVEREST II trial.[54] (Fig. 2A).

Another edge-to-edge repair system, the PASCAL Precision System (Edwards Lifesciences, Irvine, CA), received Food and Drug Administration (FDA) approval in 2022 (Fig. 2B). With the goal of improving upon some of the notable limitations experienced with the MitraClip device, the PASCAL Precision system included improved multidimensional catheter steering, independent leaflet grasping, device elongation, and a central spacer aimed to reduce complications encountered during device deployment. The CLASP II Study aimed to compare these two technologies, with 180 propensity score-matched patients and found no significant differences between them.[55] Another study found the same results, with comparable rates of device deployment success, degree of MR at discharge, and patient mortality rates. Importantly, at 1-year follow-up, there was no significant difference in the degree of MR between patients treated with MitraClip and PASCAL.[56] While these results are impressive, patients with CS were excluded from these clinical trials that established the evidence basis for TEER due to their high-risk profiles and poor outcomes.

When investigating TEER outcomes in patients with acute MR complicated by CS, it is important to note that among this population, baseline risk of mortality is extremely high, and they are often at prohibitive risk for other surgical interventions, meaning that TEER is used as a salvage therapy. TEER's innate role, therefore, presents a challenge for retrospectively analyzing absolute mortality benefit, since many patients who may be ideal candidates for TEER, elect other interventional approaches, or do not survive to TEER intervention.

There have been two large-scale studies investigating the use of TEER in patients with CS due to acute MR. In a retrospective analysis of the Centers for Medicare and Medicaid Services database, Tang and colleagues identified 38,166 individuals diagnosed with MR and CS between January 2014 and March 2019.[57] Using a propensity score matching analysis, the authors compared survival between 596 matched pairs of patients who did and did not receive TEER with MitraClip during their initial hospitalization. Patients who underwent intervention with TEER were found to have longer stays in the intensive care unit, however, they had significantly lower in-hospital (odds ratio, 0.6; 95% CI, 0.47–0.77; $P < .001$) and 1-year (hazard ratio,

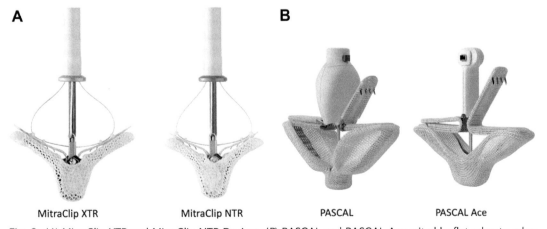

A   **B**

MitraClip XTR   MitraClip NTR   PASCAL   PASCAL Ace

Fig. 2. (A) MitraClip XTR and MitraClip NTR Devices. (B) PASCAL and PASCAL Ace mitral leaflet edge-to-edge repair devices. (Image A MitraClip is a trademark of Abbott or its related companies. Reproduced with permission of Abbott, © 2023. All rights reserved. Image B Edwards Lifesciences LLC, Irvine, CA. These images MAY NOT BE ALTERED in any way. Additionally, it should be noted that Edwards, Edwards Lifesciences, the stylized E logo, PASCAL, PASCAL Ace are trademarks of Edwards Lifesciences Corporation.)

0.76; 95% CI, 0.65–0.88; $P < .001$) mortality rates compared to their non-TEER counterparts. Though limited by its retrospective design, this study provides preliminary data suggesting that TEER may be an effective alternative to surgical intervention among high-risk patients with acute MR complicated by CS.

In another large-scale study by Simard and colleagues, 3,797 patients from the Society of Thoracic Surgeons–American College of Cardiology Transcatheter Valve Therapy (STS/ACC TVT) Registry were reviewed.[58] Data included patients with degenerative, functional, or mixed MR complicated by CS. TEER was successfully implemented in 85.6% of patients, approximately half of whom received multiple clips, adding to the difficulty of the procedure. Patients who did not achieve procedural success, due to either an unsuccessful procedure or an insignificant reduction in MR, experienced longer lengths of hospital stay, higher in-hospital mortality rates, and higher 30-day mortality rates. Procedural success was associated with a 30-day mortality rate of 34.5% compared to 55.5% in patients with unsuccessful procedures. Several complications due to TEER were highlighted in this cohort, including major bleeding, stroke, and single leaflet TEER attachment. In patients who did not achieve procedural success, higher left ventricular ejection fraction (LVEF) and lesser MR grade were reported, however, their in-hospital mortality remained higher. Similar to the results reported by Tang and colleagues, this study suggests that successful TEER may reduce mortality among high-risk patients with AMR complicated by CS—albeit—with some notable risks.[57,58]

Ideal Anatomic and Clinical Selection Criteria

A majority of patients with CS will have prohibitively high STS scores, making them unsuitable for surgical mitral valve repair/replacement. Indeed, one study showed a 22% survival rate 30-days after surgery.[59] Regrettably, this restricts the available definitive treatment choices for these patients to 1–TEER. However, specific anatomic characteristics features may present challenges given the existing range of TEER devices available. Unfavorable characteristics may include calcification within leaflet grasping zones, multi-segment pathology, active endocarditis, and coronary ischemia which may have precipitated the patient's CS. The risks associated with taking a patient to TEER when the patient's anatomy is unfavorable may outweigh any possible benefits, but it also leaves the patient without definitive treatments apart from high-risk salvage surgery. Providers may elect to move forward

with TEER when there is only a relative contraindication, since even a slight reduction of MR from severe to moderate may provide enough therapeutic benefit to stabilize the patient. In patients without CS, TEER has been found to have lower rates of in-hospital mortality when compared head-to-head with surgery.[59] As the technology continues to improve, and new devices become less reliant on patient anatomy, the mortality gap between TEER and surgery may continue to grow, as more patients become viable TEER candidates, and the selection pool for salvage surgeries shrinks further.

The development of new mechanical support options that bridge patients to definitive management may also create new factors to consider in the implementation of TEER. It will be essential to study the interactions of multiple devices in such a limited space as it may create iatrogenic anatomic incompatibility for TEER management, which could also limit the feasibility of TEER and favor surgical repair or replacement.

Patient selection continues to be one of the key hurdles in the current landscape of prospective randomized controlled trials concerning acute MR with CS. Enrolling patients in clinical trials can be a challenge in the face of emergent conditions demanding streamlined management. Furthermore, providers may be hesitant to use unfamiliar technology in time-sensitive situations when there is limited data with respect to a patient's anatomic suitability in addition to the absence of global efficacy data. These unavoidable factors can bias selection toward more stable patients who survive to the 24-h mark and are in conditions more favorable for procedural success. Predictably, this creates a bias in the literature, favoring patients with amenable anatomy and fewer comorbidities. To avoid these challenges, current studies often opt for a retrospective format, which while persuasive, must be validated by randomized controlled trials. The CAPITAL-MINOS trial will be 1 such trial, comparing the efficacy of TEER to medical therapy in acute MR patients with CS.[60] This trial is enrolling patients with advanced CS, accepting only patients who are SCAI stage C or D, at least 3+ MR, and who are unable to receive durable MCS. This study will likely fill a void in the literature and provide valuable insight into the management of critically ill patients (Table 2 and 3).

THE FUTURE OF DEFINITIVE MANAGEMENT

Several transcatheter valve replacement approaches are currently under investigation in

Table 2
Ideal patient characteristics favoring either transcatheter edge-to-edge or surgical repair/replacement

	Favorable for Transcatheter Edge-To-Edge Repair	Favorable for Surgical Repair/Replacement
Anatomic		
Calcifications	>5 mm distal leaflet tip without calcification	Extensive, severe annular calcification, calcification within grasping zone
Coaptation	Depth <11 mm and >2 mm	Depth >10 mm
Flail Gap	Flail gap <15 mm	Flail gap >15 mm
Leaflet Size	Long posterior leaflet >10 mm	Short posterior leaflet (<7 mm)
Other		Multi-segment pathology, bi-leaflet flail, small mitral valve area, multiple regurgitant jets, MR due to clefts
STS Score	>8%	<8%[a]
MV Gradient	≤5 mm Hg	>5 mm Hg
SCAI Staging	D or E	A, B, or C
Primary MR	Focal lesion with favorable flail gap	Multifocal lesion, Focal lesion with unfavorable flail gap (eg, papillary muscle rupture)
Secondary MR	Favorable Anatomy: LVEF 20%–50 LVESD < 70 mm PASP < 70 mm Hg "Disproportionate" MR	
Comorbidities	Functional MR	Coronary Ischemia
	Pulmonary HTN	Undergoing concurrent CABG
	Frailty	Lack of transseptal access
	Prior sternotomy	Chronic Rheumatic Heart Disease
	Porcelain aorta	Active Endocarditis
	Liver Cirrhosis	
	Multiorgan failure due to CS	

Abbreviations: CABG, coronary artery bypass grafting; CS, cardiogenic shock; HTN, hypertension; LVEF, left ventricular ejection fraction; LVESD, left ventricular end-systolic dimension; MR, mitral regurgitation; PASP, pulmonary artery systolic pressure.

[a] Any patient >55 y.o. presenting with MVR and CS alone will have a morbidity/mortality rate of >40% according to the STS calculator. Patients with concurrent CAD, MI, mechanical support, inotrope support, and in emergent salvage status may have morbidity/mortality rates up to 90%.

clinical trials.[61,62] They would provide an avenue for further definitive management of acute MR, especially since many cases are incompatible with a surgical approach, as previously discussed. As the toolbox for treating acute MR continues to grow, it is essential to continue reassessing our current devices for efficacy and optimization. Novel transcatheter valve replacement devices such as Tendyne (Abbott Vascular, Abbott Park, Illinois), Intrepid (Medtronic, Minneapolis, MN), and EVOQUE system (Edwards Lifesciences, Irvine, CA) aim to overcome some of the anatomic limitations of TEER repair with the MitraClip system (flail gap, etc.).

Tendyne utilizes an apical tether outside of the heart to hold a MV replacement made of three leaflets that fit over the native anatomy, in order to address either primary or secondary MR. Studies investigating the efficacy of the Tendyne system have found that at 2-years post-implantation, MR was completely resolved in 93% of patients and all-cause mortality was 39% compared with the estimated baseline mortality of 41.6%.[63] The same study found that these patients experienced significantly decreased LVEF, with a change of −5.8%, and were at risk for adverse bleeding events associated with long-term anticoagulation. The "Clinical Trial to

Table 3
Outcome data for transcatheter edge-to-edge repair (TEER) and surgical mitral valve replacement/repair

Author Year	No. of Patients	Age (Mean years)	Etiology	Intervention	Transcatheter Edge-To-Edge Repair				Surgical Mitral Valve Replacement/Repair			
					In-Hospital Mortality	1-y Mortality	Hospitalization	Procedural Success (Absolute MR Reduction ≤2+)	In-Hospital Mortality	1-y Mortality	Hospitalization	Procedural Success (Absolute MR Reduction ≤2+)
Adamo et al.[67] 2015	16	69 ± 13	Acute MR - Cardiogenic Shock	TEER only	1 (6%)	3 (19%)	8 (50%)	94% (56% reduced to 1+ MR, 38% reduced to 2+ MR)				
Haberman et al.[59] 2022	471	73 ± 11	Acute MR and Secondary MR	TEER and Surgery	6 (6%)	16 (17%)	13 (13%)	93% (Defined as MR ≤ 2+)	17 (16%)	32 (31%)	n/a	92%
Flint et al.[68] 2019	12	71.7 ± 12.8	Acute MR Cardiogenic Shock	TEER	1 (8%)	30 d: 2 (17%)	N/a	100%				
Simard et al.[58] 2022	3249	73 ± 11	Acute and Secondary MR Cardiogenic Shock	TEER	296 (9.1%)	1124 (34.6%)	962 (29.6%)	88.20%				
Jung et al.[69] 2021	141	68.9 ± 12.1	Acute MR Cardiogenic Shock (Not eligible for surgery)	TEER	22 (15.6%)	55 (42.6%)	26 (18.4%)	88.70%				
Cheng et al.[70] 2019	29	65.5 ± 17	Acute MR Cardiogenic Shock	TEER	4 (14%)	6 mo: 7 (25%)		90%				
Estevez Loureiro et al.[71] 2021	93	70.3 ± 10.2	MR after Acute Myocardial Infarction in Cardiogenic Shock	TEER		30 d: 5 (10%)	3 mo: 13 7 mo mortality: 16%	90%				
Stone et al.[72] (COAPT) 2018 2023 (5-y Follow Up)	302	71.7 ± 11.8	Moderate-to-severe MR with Heart Failure	TEER		30 d: 2.3 5 y: 57.3%	5 y: 77%	95%				

| Lorusso et al.[50] 2008 | 279 | 62 ± 14 | Acute MR Cardiogenic Shock | Surgery | 30 d: 22.5 15-y survival: 67 ± 10% | Pts with MI: 27.4 Pts with Degenerative MV Disease: 16.6 Pts with Acute Endocarditis: 21.8% |

Abbreviations: MR, mitral regurgitation; TEER, transcatheter edge-to-edge repair

Evaluate the Safety and Effectiveness of Using the Tendyne Transcatheter Mitral Valve System for the Treatment of Symptomatic Mitral Regurgitation" (SUMMIT) is a randomized controlled trial, comparing the Tendyne system to the widely used MitraClip.[61] This study is slated to conclude in June 2027.

Another novel device, the Intrepid, also tackles secondary MR by deploying a self-expanding stent anchored by a flexible brim around the mitral annulus via a transseptal approach. An early feasibility study in 15 patients found that at 30-days, there was complete reduction of MR. In that same study, 6 out of 15 patients also experienced major hematological events, usually at the access site, but there were no deaths, strokes, or reinterventions.[62] The Intrepid system is currently being tested in a non-randomized controlled trial called "Transcatheter Mitral Valve Replacement With the Medtronic Intrepid TMVR System in Patients with Severe Symptomatic Mitral Regurgitation" (APOLLO), with an estimated completion date of October 2028.[64]

The transcatheter, transseptal EVOQUE system was used to treat functional, degenerative, and mixed MR in a first-in-human experience of 14 patients, where it was found to reduce MR to mild or none in approximately 93% of patients. Adverse outcomes at 30 days included 1 non-cardiovascular mortality (7.1%), 2 strokes (14.3%), no myocardial infarctions, and no rehospitalizations.[65] The valve consists of a self-expanding frame, bovine pericardial leaflets, and a fabric skirt to minimize paravalvular leak. The valve has a unique anchoring mechanism to use the annulus, leaflets, and chords for secure placement in the anatomy. Investigation of the next-generation EVOQUE Eos system is underway.[66]

As these clinical trials begin to produce results, it is important to note that many specifically exclude patients with CS for their trials. This means that the timeline for CS patients is greatly elongated, even though they represent some of the highest risk patients who may benefit the most from these novel technologies. As investigation into the feasibility and applicability of these transcatheter-based approaches continues to grow, patient inclusion criteria will expand, paving the way for novel non-surgical interventions in CS.

SUMMARY

In conclusion, the management of acute MR complicated by CS is a complex and challenging task. Early identification and risk stratification of patients with acute MR and CS is crucial, and the integration of invasive hemodynamic monitoring is essential in guiding therapeutic strategies. Afterload reduction with systemic vasodilators, particularly nitroprusside, plays a pivotal role in optimizing hemodynamics and minimizing regurgitant fraction. Temporary mechanical circulatory support devices, such as IABP and Impella-CP, offer valuable options in stabilizing patients and bridging them to definitive management.

TEER with devices like MitraClip and PASCAL provides a promising alternative for patients at high surgical risk. Despite challenges in patient selection and anatomic suitability, retrospective studies indicate that successful TEER might reduce mortality rates among high-risk patients with acute MR and CS. Ongoing clinical trials and the emergence of novel transcatheter valve replacement approaches, such as Tendyne, Intrepid, and EVOQUE, present exciting prospects for the future of MR management.

However, the landscape of acute MR and CS management is continuously evolving. As newer technologies and approaches emerge, addressing the specific needs of critically ill patients, refining patient selection criteria, and conducting rigorous clinical trials will be essential. By integrating these advancements with comprehensive patient care and multidisciplinary collaboration, clinicians can offer more effective and tailored interventions, ultimately improving outcomes for this challenging patient population.

CLINICS CARE POINTS

- Early recognition and risk stratification is essential in the management of mitral regurgitation complicated by cardiogenic shock.
- Initial management should focus on hemodynamic stabilization through the use of pharmacotherapy and potentially mechanical circulatory support devices to optimize cardiac output and perfusion.
- Multi-disciplinary collaboration between interventional cardiology, cardiac surgery, and heart failure specialists is essential to optimize patient care prior to definitive management and to determine the optimal definitive management strategy for each patient.

DISCLOSURE

The authors have nothing to disclose.

REFERENCES

1. Jung RG, Di Santo P, Mathew R, et al. implications of myocardial infarction on management and outcome in cardiogenic shock. J Am Heart Assoc 2021;10:e021570.
2. Di Santo P, Mathew R, Jung RG, et al. Impact of baseline beta-blocker use on inotrope response and clinical outcomes in cardiogenic shock: a subgroup analysis of the DOREMI trial. Crit Care 2021; 25:289.
3. Thiele H, Ohman EM, de Waha-Thiele S, et al. Management of cardiogenic shock complicating myocardial infarction: an update 2019. Eur Heart J 2019;40:2671–83.
4. Douedi S, Douedi H. Mitral Regurgitation. [Updated 2023 Apr 7]. In: StatPearls [Internet]. Treasure Island (FL): StatPearls Publishing; 2023. Available at: https://www.ncbi.nlm.nih.gov/books/NBK553135/.
5. Otto CM, Nishimura RA, Bonow RO, et al. 2020 ACC/AHA guideline for the management of patients with valvular heart disease: executive summary: a report of the american college of cardiology/american heart association joint committee on clinical practice guidelines. Circulation 2021;143:e35–71.
6. Goldstein D, Moskowitz AJ, Gelijns AC, et al. Two-year outcomes of surgical treatment of severe ischemic mitral regurgitation. N Engl J Med 2016; 374:344–53.
7. Libby P, Bonow RO, Mann DL, et al. Braunwald's heart disease: a textbook of cardiovascular medicine. Philadelphia, PA: Elsevier Science; 2021.
8. Stout KK, Verrier ED. Acute valvular regurgitation. Circulation 2009;119:3232–41.
9. Roberts WC, Braunwald E, Morrow AG. Acute severe mitral regurgitation secondary to ruptured chordae tendineae: clinical, hemodynamic, and pathologic considerations. Circulation 1966;33: 58–70.
10. Kapur NK, Kanwar M, Sinha SS, et al. Criteria for defining stages of cardiogenic shock severity. J Am Coll Cardiol 2022;80:185–98.
11. Naidu SS, Baran DA, Jentzer JC, et al. SCAI SHOCK stage classification expert consensus update: A review and incorporation of validation studies. Catheter Cardiovasc Interv 2022;1:100008.
12. Basir MB, Schreiber TL, Grines CL, et al. Effect of early initiation of mechanical circulatory support on survival in cardiogenic shock. Am J Cardiol 2017;119:845–51.
13. Basir MB, Kapur NK, Patel K, et al. Improved outcomes associated with the use of shock protocols: updates from the national cardiogenic shock initiative. Catheter Cardiovasc Interv 2019;93:1173–83.

14. Tehrani BN, Truesdell AG, Psotka MA, et al. A standardized and comprehensive approach to the management of cardiogenic shock. JACC Heart Fail 2020;8:879–91.

15. Kolte D, Khera S, Aronow WS, et al. Trends in incidence, management, and outcomes of cardiogenic shock complicating ST-elevation myocardial infarction in the United States. J Am Heart Assoc 2014;3: e000590.

16. Gore JM, Goldberg RJ, Spodick DH, et al. A community-wide assessment of the use of pulmonary artery catheters in patients with acute myocardial infarction. Chest 1987;92:721–7.

17. Garan AR, Kanwar M, Thayer KL, et al. Complete hemodynamic profiling with pulmonary artery catheters in cardiogenic shock is associated with lower in-hospital mortality. JACC Heart Fail 2020;8: 903–13.

18. Rossello X, Vila M, Rivas-Lasarte M, et al. Impact of pulmonary artery catheter use on short- and long-term mortality in patients with cardiogenic shock. Cardiology 2017;136:61–9.

19. Vahanian A, Beyersdorf F, Praz F, et al. 2021 ESC/ EACTS Guidelines for the management of valvular heart disease. Eur Heart J 2022;43:561–632.

20. Stamm C, Friehs I, Cowan DB, et al. Dopamine treatment of postischemic contractile dysfunction rapidly induces calcium-dependent pro-apoptotic signaling. Circulation 2002;106:I290–8.

21. Basir MB, Lemor A, Gorgis S, et al. Vasopressors independently associated with mortality in acute myocardial infarction and cardiogenic shock. Catheter Cardiovasc Interv 2022;99:650–7.

22. Baran DA, Grines CL, Bailey S, et al. SCAI clinical expert consensus statement on the classification of cardiogenic shock: This document was endorsed by the American College of Cardiology (ACC), the American Heart Association (AHA), the Society of Critical Care Medicine (SCCM), and the Society of Thoracic Surgeons (STS) in April 2019. Catheter Cardiovasc Interv 2019;94:29–37.

23. Otto CM, Nishimura RA, Bonow RO, et al. 2020 ACC/AHA guideline for the management of patients with valvular heart disease: a report of the american college of cardiology/american heart association joint committee on clinical practice guidelines. Circulation 2021;143:e72–227.

24. Goodman DJ, Rossen RM, Holloway EL, et al. Effect of nitroprusside on left ventricular dynamics in mitral regurgitation. Circulation 1974;50:1025–32.

25. Mullens W, Abrahams Z, Francis GS, et al. Sodium nitroprusside for advanced low-output heart failure. J Am Coll Cardiol 2008;52:200–7.

26. Chatterjee K, Parmley WW, Swan HJ, et al. Beneficial effects of vasodilator agents in severe mitral regurgitation due to dysfunction of subvalvar apparatus. Circulation 1973;48:684–90.

27. Horstkotte D, Schulte HD, Niehues R, et al. Diagnostic and therapeutic considerations in acute, severe mitral regurgitation: experience in 42 consecutive patients entering the intensive care unit with pulmonary edema. J Heart Valve Dis 1993;2:512–22.

28. Nessim SJ, Richardson RMA. Dialysis for thiocyanate intoxication: a case report and review of the literature. ASAIO J 2006;52:479–81.

29. Cohn JN, Burke LP. Nitroprusside. Ann Intern Med 1979;91:752–7.

30. Aroney CN, Semigran MJ, Dec GW, et al. Inotropic effect of nicardipine in patients with heart failure: assessment by left ventricular end-systolic pressure-volume analysis. J Am Coll Cardiol 1989;14: 1331–8.

31. Nordlander M, Sjöquist P-O, Ericsson H, et al. Pharmacodynamic, pharmacokinetic and clinical effects of clevidipine, an ultrashort-acting calcium antagonist for rapid blood pressure control. Cardiovasc Drug Rev 2004;22:227–50.

32. Bhardwaj B, Sidhu G, Balla S, et al. Outcomes and hospital utilization in patients with papillary muscle rupture associated with acute myocardial infarction. Am J Cardiol 2020;125:1020–5.

33. Pahuja M, Singh M, Patel A, et al. Utilization of mechanical circulatory support devices in chordae tendinae and papillary muscle rupture complicating st-elevation myocardial infarction: insights from nationwide inpatient sample. J Am Coll Cardiol 2018;71:A219.

34. Damluji AA, Van Diepen S, Katz JN, et al. mechanical complications of acute myocardial infarction: a scientific statement from the american heart association. Circulation 2021;144:E16–35.

35. Thiele H, Zeymer U, Thelemann N, et al. intraaortic balloon pump in cardiogenic shock complicating acute myocardial infarction. Circulation 2019;139: 395–403.

36. Baldetti L, Pagnesi M, Gramegna M, et al. Intra-aortic balloon pumping in acute decompensated heart failure with hypoperfusion: from pathophysiology to clinical practice. Circulation Heart failure 2021;14:e008527.

37. Dekker ALAJ, Reesink KD, van der Veen FH, et al. Intra-aortic balloon pumping in acute mitral regurgitation reduces aortic impedance and regurgitant fraction. Shock 2003;19:334–8.

38. Kettner J, Sramko M, Holek M, et al. Utility of intra-aortic balloon pump support for ventricular septal rupture and acute mitral regurgitation complicating acute myocardial infarction. Am J Cardiol 2013;112: 1709–13.

39. Jalil B, El-Kersh K, Frizzell J, et al. Impella percutaneous left ventricular assist device for severe acute ischaemic mitral regurgitation as a bridge to surgery. BMJ Case Rep 2017;2017:1–4.

40. Vandenbriele C, Balthazar T, Wilson J, et al. Left Impella®-device as bridge from cardiogenic shock with acute, severe mitral regurgitation to MitraClip®-procedure: a new option for critically ill patients. Eur Heart J Acute Cardiovasc Care 2021;10:415–21.

41. Takagi K, Shojima T, Kono T, et al. ECPELLA as the bridge to surgery in patients with cardiogenic shock due to post-infarct papillary muscle rupture: management of mechanical circulatory support during operation. J Artif Organs 2023;26:237–41.

42. Kawanami S, Egami Y, Nishino M, et al. One-week Impella CP support for papillary muscle rupture as a bridge to surgery: a case report. Eur Heart J Case Rep 2023;7:ytad274.

43. DiVita M, Visveswaran GK, Makam K, et al. Emergent tandemheart-ECMOfor acute severe mitral regurgitation with cardiogenic shock and hypoxaemia: a case series. European Heart Journal - Case Reports 2021;4:1–6.

44. Matteucci M, Fina D, Jiritano F, et al. The use of extracorporeal membrane oxygenation in the setting of postinfarction mechanical complications: outcome analysis of the extracorporeal life support organization registry. Interact Cardiovasc Thorac Surg 2020;31:369–74.

45. Cheng R, Hachamovitch R, Kittleson M, et al. Complications of extracorporeal membrane oxygenation for treatment of cardiogenic shock and cardiac arrest: a meta-analysis of 1,866 adult patients. Ann Thorac Surg 2014;97:610–6.

46. Juo Y-Y, Skancke M, Sanaiha Y, et al. Efficacy of distal perfusion cannulae in preventing limb ischemia during extracorporeal membrane oxygenation: a systematic review and meta-analysis. Artif Organs 2017;41:E263–73.

47. Marbach JA, Faugno AJ, Pacifici S, et al. Strategies to reduce limb ischemia in peripheral venoarterial extracorporeal membrane oxygenation: A systematic review and Meta-analysis. Int J Cardiol 2022; 361:77–84.

48. Ekanem E, Gattani R, Bakhshi H, et al. Combined venoarterial ECMO and impella-cp circulatory support for cardiogenic shock due to papillary muscle rupture. JACC (J Am Coll Cardiol): Case Reports 2020;2:2169–72.

49. Staudacher DL, Bode C, Wengenmayer T. Severe mitral regurgitation requiring ECMO therapy treated by interventional valve reconstruction using the MitraClip. Catheter Cardiovasc Interv 2015;85:170–5.

50. Lorusso R, Gelsomino S, De Cicco G, et al. Mitral valve surgery in emergency for severe acute regurgitation: analysis of postoperative results from a multicentre study. Eur J Cardio Thorac Surg 2008; 33:573–82.

51. Thompson Christopher R, Buller Christopher E, Sleeper Lynn A, et al. Cardiogenic shock due to acute severe mitral regurgitation complicating acute myocardial infarction: a report from the SHOCK Trial Registry. J Am Coll Cardiol 2000;36: 1104–9.

52. Feldman T, Foster E, Glower DD, et al. Percutaneous repair or surgery for mitral regurgitation. N Engl J Med 2011;364:1395–406.

53. Mack MJ, Lindenfeld J, Abraham WT, et al. 3-year outcomes of transcatheter mitral valve repair in patients with heart failure. J Am Coll Cardiol 2021;77: 1029–40.

54. Sodhi N, Asch FM, Ruf T, et al. Clinical outcomes with transcatheter edge-to-edge repair in atrial functional MR from the EXPAND study. JACC Cardiovasc Interv 2022;15:1723–30.

55. Lim DS, Smith RL, Gillam LD, et al. Randomized comparison of transcatheter edge-to-edge repair for degenerative mitral regurgitation in prohibitive surgical risk patients. JACC Cardiovasc Interv 2022; 15:2523–36.

56. Schneider L, Markovic S, Mueller K, et al. Mitral valve transcatheter edge-to-edge repair using mitraclip or PASCAL: a multicenter propensity score-matched comparison. JACC Cardiovasc Interv 2022;15:2554–67.

57. Tang GHL, Estevez-Loureiro R, Yu Y, et al. survival following edge-to-edge transcatheter mitral valve repair in patients with cardiogenic shock: a nationwide analysis. J Am Heart Assoc 2021;10:e019882.

58. Simard T, Vemulapalli S, Jung RG, et al. Transcatheter edge-to-edge mitral valve repair in patients with severe mitral regurgitation and cardiogenic shock. J Am Coll Cardiol 2022;80:2072–84.

59. Haberman D, Estévez-Loureiro R, Benito-Gonzalez T, et al. Conservative, surgical, and percutaneous treatment for mitral regurgitation shortly after acute myocardial infarction. Eur Heart J 2022;43: 641–50.

60. Parlow S, Di Santo P, Jung RG, et al. Transcatheter mitral valve repair for inotrope dependent cardiogenic shock - Design and rationale of the CAPITAL MINOS trial. Am Heart J 2022;254:81–7.

61. Anon. Clinical Trial to Evaluate the Safety and Effectiveness of Using the Tendyne Transcatheter Mitral Valve System for the Treatment of Symptomatic Mitral Regurgitation - Full Text View - Clinicaltrials.gov. https://classic.clinicaltrials.gov/ct2/show/ NCT03433274. Accessed July 25, 2023.

62. Zahr F, Song HK, Chadderdon SM, et al. 30-day outcomes following transfemoral transseptal transcatheter mitral valve replacement: intrepid TMVR early feasibility study results. JACC Cardiovasc Interv 2022;15:80–9.

63. Muller DWM, Sorajja P, Duncan A, et al. 2-year outcomes of transcatheter mitral valve replacement in patients with severe symptomatic mitral regurgitation. J Am Coll Cardiol 2021;78:1847–59.

64. Anon. Transcatheter Mitral Valve Replacement With the Medtronic IntrepidTM TMVR System in Patients With Severe Symptomatic Mitral Regurgitation. - Full Text View - Clinicaltrials.gov. https://classic.clinicaltrials.gov/ct2/show/NCT03242642. Accessed July 25, 2023.

65. Webb J, Hensey M, Fam N, et al. Transcatheter mitral valve replacement with the transseptal EVOQUE system. JACC Cardiovasc Interv 2020;13:2418–26.

66. Anon. Edwards EVOQUE Eos MISCEND Study. https://classic.clinicaltrials.gov/ct2/show/NCT02718001. Accessed July 25, 2023.

67. Adamo M, Barbanti M, Curello S, et al. Effectiveness of mitraclip therapy in patients with refractory heart failure. J Interv Cardiol 2015;28:61–8.

68. Flint K, Brieke A, Wiktor D, et al. Percutaneous edge-to-edge mitral valve repair may rescue select patients in cardiogenic shock: Findings from a single center case series. Catheter Cardiovasc Interv 2019;94:E82–7.

69. Jung RG, Simard T, Kovach C, et al. Transcatheter mitral valve repair in cardiogenic shock and mitral regurgitation: a patient-level, multicenter analysis. JACC Cardiovasc Interv 2021;14:1–11.

70. Cheng R, Dawkins S, Hamilton MA, et al. Percutaneous mitral repair for patients in cardiogenic shock requiring inotropes and temporary mechanical circulatory support. JACC Cardiovasc Interv 2019;12:2440–1.

71. Estévez-Loureiro R, Shuvy M, Taramasso M, et al. Use of MitraClip for mitral valve repair in patients with acute mitral regurgitation following acute myocardial infarction: Effect of cardiogenic shock on outcomes (IREMMI Registry). Catheter Cardiovasc Interv 2021;97:1259–67.

72. Stone GW, Lindenfeld J, Abraham WT, et al. transcatheter mitral-valve repair in patients with heart failure. N Engl J Med 2018;379:2307–18.

Postsurgical Transcatheter Mitral Valve Replacement

Faraj Kargoli, MD, MPH[a], Abdullah K. Al Qaraghuli, MD[b], Hao Kenith Fang, MD[c], Marvin H. Eng, MD[d],*

KEYWORDS

- Transcatheter mitral valve replacement • Surgical mitral valve replacement • Mitral valve
- Valvular heart disease • Valve in ring • Valve in valve

KEY POINTS

- Reintervention is commonly required postsurgical mitral valve replacement (SMVR) or repair due to bioprosthetic valve and annuloplasty ring degeneration. However, redo SMVR is associated with a high risk of morbidity and mortality.
- Postsurgical transcatheter mitral valve replacement (TMVR) is a safe and less-invasive alternative that has repeatedly been shown to be associated with improved survival and lower rates of complications compared with redo SMVR.
- Comprehensive patient evaluation and thorough procedural planning are key to successful TMVR.

INTRODUCTION

Mitral regurgitation (MR) is the most common valvular abnormality, affecting approximately 24.2 million people worldwide.[1] Surgical treatment, specifically surgical mitral valve repair or replacement (SMVR), remains the standard of care for the treatment of MR. The use of bioprosthetic valves has been increasingly favored over mechanical valves in the past 2 decades, due to the lower risk of thrombotic complications and avoidance of anticoagulation.[2] However, evidence suggests that the bioprosthetic valves used in SMVR show signs of structural deterioration within 15 years in nearly half of patients, often necessitating reintervention.[3,4] Although surgical outcomes have improved, redo SMVR still carries higher risks of morbidity and mortality compared with primary SMVR, with mortality rates exceeding 30% at 5 years.[3,5] Therefore, transcatheter mitral valve replacement (TMVR) has emerged as a less-invasive

and promising alternative therapy to mitigate surgical risk for these patients. Specifically, the Sapien family of balloon-expandable valves (Edwards Lifesciences, Irvine, CA) has gained significant traction in performing mitral valve-in-valve (MViV) and mitral valve-in-ring (MViR) procedures. This review highlights some key aspects of MViV and MViR, with a focus on appropriate patient selection, procedural planning, potential challenges, as well as outcomes for postsurgical TMVR.

ANATOMIC CHALLENGES OF TRANSCATHETER MITRAL VALVE REPLACEMENT

The widespread uptake and procedural success rates of transcatheter aortic valve replacement (TAVR) have prompted investigators to further explore the potential utility of TMVR as an alternative to SMVR.[6] However, the complex anatomy and hemodynamics of the mitral valve

[a] Division of Cardiology, University of Arizona, Banner University Medical Center, 1111 East McDowell Road, Phoenix, AZ 85006, USA; [b] MedStar Health Research Institute, MedStar Washington Hospital Center, 110 Irving Street Northwest, Washington, DC 20010, USA; [c] Division of Cardiothoracic Surgery, Banner University Medical Center, 1111 East McDowell Road, Phoenix, AZ 85006, USA; [d] Structural Heart Program, University of Arizona, Banner University Medical Center, 755 East McDowell Road, Phoenix, AZ 85006, USA
* Corresponding author.
E-mail address: marvin.eng@bannerhealth.com

Intervent Cardiol Clin 13 (2024) 207–216
https://doi.org/10.1016/j.iccl.2023.12.002
2211-7458/24/© 2023 Elsevier Inc. All rights reserved.

make TMVR a far more challenging procedure than TAVR, be it on a native or a failed bio-prosthetic valve. The native mitral valve is a dynamic three-dimensional (3D) system that has an additional subvalvular component. The valve consists of the saddle-shaped rigid annulus, as well as the anterior and posterior mitral valve leaflets. These leaflets are attached to the collagenous chordae tendineae that bulge from the papillary muscles forming the subvalvular apparatus. Given the multiple substrates comprising the mitral valve, its asymmetric D-shape configuration, and the dynamic annular region with limited rigidity, a variety of complex anchoring techniques are often required for valve fixation in native TMVR.[6,7] Additionally, its position relative to the left ventricular outflow tract (LVOT) renders LVOT obstruction (LVOTO) a serious risk that requires antecedent accounting and mitigation planning.[7]

Despite the aforementioned challenges, TMVR remains an appealing alternative to redo SMVR. In a recently published meta-analysis of 9 retrospective cohort studies encompassing data from 3038 patients, TMVR (MViV or MViR) was associated with lower rates of in-hospital mortality (OR: 0.44, 95% CI: 0.30, 0.64, $P < .001$), stroke (OR 0.44, 95% CI: 0.29, 0.67, $P < .001$), and vascular complications (OR: 0.58, 95% CI 0.43, 0.78, $P = .004$) compared with redo SMVR.[8] This is particularly important to note, given that patients undergoing TMVR tended to be older and with significantly higher Society of Thoracic Surgeons (STS) scores compared with those who underwent redo SMVR.[8] Table 1 summarizes the currently available data on MViV, MViR, and SMVR outcomes.

MITRAL VALVE-IN-VALVE VERSUS REDO SURGICAL MITRAL VALVE REPLACEMENT OUTCOMES

MViV gained Food and Drug Administration approval in 2017 and has demonstrated superiority over redo SMVR in several studies since. In the largest and most recent analysis of 4243 patients from the Transcatheter Valve Therapy (TVT) registry, MViV had an implant success rate of 97% and was associated with effective and durable reduction in MR, whereby 87% of patients had no evidence of MR at 1 year follow-up (unpublished data).[9] In addition, a 43% drop in mean gradient was observed on echocardiography at 1-year follow-up (Table 2).[9] Similarly, analysis of data from 2550 patients from the Nationwide Inpatient Sample database found that patients who underwent MViV had a significantly lower rate of in-hospital mortality compared with redo-SMVR (2.5% vs 7.6%, respectively, $P = .001$), despite being an older cohort with a higher burden of comorbidity.[10] Patients who underwent MViV were also more likely to be discharged home (64.6% vs 20.3%), have shorter lengths of stay (3 days vs 10 days), and less frequent complications, such as acute kidney injury (13.9% vs 36.7%) or pneumonia (<2.8% vs 10.1%) compared with those who underwent redo SMVR.[10] Another meta-analysis of 6 retrospective cohort studies (n = 707 patients) similarly supports the use of MViV over redo SMVR because they found that patients who underwent MViV had lower rates of complications, shorter hospital lengths of stay, and similar 30-day mortality rates, despite being older in age and with more comorbidities than those who underwent redo SMVR.[11]

PATIENT EVALUATION FOR POST-SURGICAL MITRAL VALVE-IN-VALVE

Before proceeding with TMVR, it is imperative that the operator thoroughly evaluates patients to confirm their eligibility for TMVR and complete comprehensive preoperative planning to maximize success rates. A heart team evaluation is necessary to evaluate surgical candidacy and review the risks and benefits of proceeding with either TMVR or redo SMVR, considering the patient's age, comorbidities, and STS score.

Advances in multimodality imaging have rendered cardiovascular imaging crucial in the diagnosis, preprocedural planning, procedural guidance, and follow-up of TMVR therapies.[12]

Noninvasive transthoracic and transesophageal echocardiography are typically used first as a method of characterizing the mitral valve, assessing for the severity of MR, as well as identifying the potential for concurrent mitral stenosis or tricuspid regurgitation.[13] The echocardiogram also allows for the identification of possible contraindications to TMVR or factors that may complicate the intervention, such as the presence of infective endocarditis, intracardiac thrombus, or paravalvular leak (PVL).[13] Cardiac computed tomography (CCT) is then used as a noninvasive imaging technique with high isotropic submillimeter spatial resolution, which provides high accuracy for characterization of the bioprosthesis and 3D procedural simulation (Fig. 1).[14] The CCT yields detailed information regarding the dimensions of the mitral annulus and provides an assessment of the risk for LVOTO, by allowing for neo-LVOT measurement after the simulated

Table 1
Mitral valve-in-valve and valve-in-ring outcomes and procedural complications

	Simonato et al,[18] 2021. VIV	Yoon et al,[25] 2019. VIV	Guerreo et al. VIV	Whisenant et al,[17] 2020. VIV	Simonato et al,[21] 2021. VIR	Yoon et al,[34]. VIR	Guerreo et al VIR.	Goel et al,[9] 2023. VIV
N	857	322	680	1529	222	141	123	4243
Technical success (%)	93.5	94.4	90.9	96.8	81.5	80.9	82.9	96.6
In-hospital Mortality (%)	2.1	…	…	4	0.5	…	…	3.2
30-d mortality (%)	6.5	6.2	8.1	5.4	8.6	9.9	11.5	4.3
1-y mortality (%)	13.8	14	…	16.7	23.2	30.6	…	13.4
Ventricular perforation (%)	…	1.2	1.9	1.1	…	0	2.4	0.9
LVOTO (%)	1.8	2.2	0.7	0.9	5.9	5	4.9	0.4
Valve embolization (%)	2.4	0.9	0.1	0.3	7	1.4	2.4	0.6
Second valve	2.8	2.5	1.5	…	10.1	12.1	7.3	…
Stroke (%)	1.4	2.3	1.6	0.7	…	0	1.6	4.9
Major or life-threatening bleeding (%)	8.8	6.9	9.7	…	4.7	10.6	10.4	…
Vascular complication (%)	3.2	1.6	2.9	…	0.5	3.8	4.9	4.3
AKI (%)	8.8	4.6	…	…	13	9.7	…	…
≥2+ mitral regurgitation (%)	3.1	5.6	3.6	…	16.6	18.4	13	0.8
PVL repair (%)	…	…	…	…	…	7.8	…	…

implantation of a transcatheter heart valve (THV). CCT may also help to select the most suitable location for transseptal or transapical puncture site.[12,13]

MITRAL VALVE-IN-VALVE ACCESS AND DELIVERY

Transapical access was the first described method for TMVR, although transseptal access has been increasingly used given it is less invasive and avoids the need for thoracotomy.[15,16] The transapical approach may be appealing because it offers the operator improved control over the placement of large-bore delivery sheaths as well as the coaxial alignment of the prosthesis relative to the mitral annulus. This is difficult to achieve with the transseptal approach because the operator must maneuver the delivery system at a nearly right-angle bend between the interatrial septum and mitral valve annular plane to cross the mitral valve. The transseptal approach also increases the risk of requiring

future repair of the iatrogenic atrial septal defect. Despite being a more challenging procedure, however, data from the TVT-STS registry found that among a sample of 1529 patients who underwent MViV, transseptal access was associated with shorter lengths of hospital stay (2 vs 6 days, respectively, $P < .001$) and lower 1-year all-cause mortality (15.8% vs 21.7%, respectively, $P = .03$) compared with transapical access.[17] There was no difference in the rate of in-hospital complications.[17]

Degenerated surgical valves are generally good substrates for THV anchoring. Despite the somewhat stereotypical design of surgical mitral valves, details regarding the make and size of the degenerated prosthesis are key details necessary for successful procedures. Furthermore, understanding the indication for the initial surgery (ie, endocarditis) and additional surgical procedures (ie, LVOT enlargement in double valve surgery) are important for success. With the available of surgical prosthesis details, sizing of THV is more precise and a

Table 2
Mitral valve-in-valve and mitral valve-in-ring echocardiographic follow-up

	Simonato et al,[18] 2021. VIV	Yoon et al,[25] 2019. VIV	Guerreo et al,[35] 2020. VIV	Whisenant et al,[17] 2020	Simonato et al,[21] 2021. VIR	Yoon et al,[34] 2019 VIR	Guerreo et al VIR.	Goel et al,[9] 2023. VIV
30-d mean gradient (mm Hg)	*5.6 ± 2.7	*5.9 ± 2.8	4	7.3	*6.2 ± 2.8	*6.7 ± 3.1	*4	7.6
30-d ≥2+MR (%)	*2.9	*5.6	3.6	...	*13.1	*18.4	*13	0.8
1-y mean gradient (mm Hg)	6.9 ± 3	...	...	7.0	6.7 ± 2.8	...	...	7.4
1-y ≥2+ MR (%)	5.3	...	...	...	18.3	...	...	0.9

combination of operative reports and CCT measurements should be used for THV sizing choice. It should be noted that porcine valves typically have smaller internal diameters for each labeled prosthesis size compared with bovine pericardial valves. Additionally, porcine valve leaflets do not reach the ventricular end of the posts of the surgical valves, therefore their risk for LVOT obstruction is less than that of bovine pericardial valves. Additionally, should an implanted THV required postdilation for expansion, it should be noted that some valves cannot expand due to the metal in the sewing frame (ie, Hancock, Medtronic, St. Paul, MN).

Transseptal TMVR has previously been described.[14] In brief, an arterial femoral sheath is inserted for continuous arterial pressure monitoring and a venous sheath is used for placing the temporary right ventricular pacing lead. If there is concern for LVOT obstruction, one can perform simultaneous LV and aortic hemodynamic monitoring with a dual lumen catheter or catheter/sheath combination. The right femoral vein is usually used for transseptal access. A midposterior puncture of the interatrial septum approximately 3 to 3.5 cm above the mitral annular plane is optimal (Fig. 2). After the transseptal sheath penetrates the left atrium, the sheath is exchanged for a deflectable sheath so as to allow the operator to navigate the catheter across the mitral valve into the ventricle, at which point a stiff, preformed wire can be introduced.[14] Afterward, a 12 to 14 mm balloon septostomy is performed to facilitate the passage of

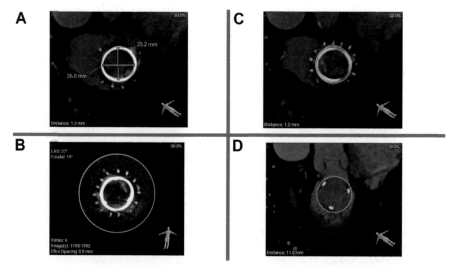

Fig. 1. MViV CCT analysis. (A, B) Sizing of 25 mm Magna valve. (C, D) Virtual simulation of 26 mm THV.

the valve across the atrial septum. The balloon can also be used to test the trajectory of the valve's delivery. The valve is typically delivered through the e-sheath (Edwards Lifesciences, Irvine, CA). Alignment of the THV to the mitral bioprosthesis is necessary to provide stable anchoring without having an excessive atrial position. Finally, to minimize stroke volume and allow for a stable THV deployment, rapid pacing is performed.[14]

PATIENT EVALUATION FOR MITRAL VALVE-IN-RING

Similar to the evaluation of patients for MViV, patients undergoing MViR should undergo transthoracic and transesophageal echocardiography, as well as CCT to gain an understanding of the ring morphology and allow for comprehensive preprocedural analysis and planning. Imaging is required to determine the THV anchoring platform, projected coaxial alignment, valve sizing, projected neo-LVOT and potential for neo-LVOT modification. It is important to note that many different rings exist, and not all rings are amenable to MViR. Additionally, we may not always encounter the classic known shape of the ring because it may have been modified by the surgeon to fit a patient's anatomy or may have been distorted over time by cardiac remodeling.[18] As such, it is often necessary to refer back to the initial operative reports or valve manufacturer to gather details on the specific ring used.

Operators should be familiar with the spectrum of rings and the differences in their shape, composition, and rigidity because it may affect procedural planning. The rings are typically "D" shaped to mimic the natural structure of the mitral annulus, and they can be complete or partial. They are composed of silicone, metal titanium cores, layered polyester, or Elgiloy, and they are classified as being rigid, semirigid, or flexible.[19,20] Analysis of data from the VIVID Registry of 1079 patients undergoing MViR found that there was no statistically significant difference in clinical outcomes at 4-year follow-up based on the type of ring used.[21]

Important factors that need to be assessed include the ring's ability to become circular, its ability to provide a good anchor, and the ring size. If a ring cannot become circular, the THV may be underexpanded or deformed, resulting in suboptimal outcomes. As such, complete rigid rings and incomplete rings make for less than ideal THV platforms.[20,22] The ability of the ring to anchor the THV is usually dependent on its

flexibility and dimensions. Although complete rigid rings are good anchors, they cannot become circular. As such, semirigid rings provide the ideal balance of being able to become circular and provide a good anchor. Ring size and dimension, such as commissure-to-commissure length, lateral-septal length area, and perimeter also need to be elicited to confirm suitability for MViR, and one may need to refer to the manufacturer's label or MViV app. Very small rings (eg, 26 mm) or large rings (eg, >34 mm) are not usually suitable for MViR.[20,22] Moreover, coaxial alignment is crucial to successful MViR implantation, and CCT is instrumental for identifying the ideal transseptal puncture site that can provide the most optimal coaxial trajectory. In some instances, the use of a periapical access may be necessary for achieving coaxial alignment (**Fig. 3** MViR images).[23]

MITRAL VALVE-IN-RING ACCESS AND DELIVERY

Transseptal MViR technique shares similarities with MViV but has specific considerations. It is a more challenging procedure with higher rates of complications such as LVOTO and PVL. A major factor contributing to this is the short landing zone afforded by the THV, thus making coaxial trajectory of paramount importance to achieve a good annular seal and mitigate PVL risk. This is likely a major factor contributing to the relatively high requirement for second valve deployment, in approximately 38.1% of cases.[24] Transseptal access makes alignment even more difficult to achieve. In some instances, the operator may consider adjusting the wire and applying catheter pressure simultaneously to improve coaxial positioning. Rapid pacing is used when deploying the THV. It is advisable to deploy the THV with a ventricular bias and using a slow 2-step inflation.[22,24]

MITIGATING LEFT VENTRICULAR OUTFLOW TRACT OBSTRUCTION RISK

LVOTO is a devastating complication of TMVR, particularly following MViR, and it is associated with a nearly 3-fold increased hazard of mortality.[25] This is due to the fact that the native anterior mitral valve or prosthetic leaflet is displaced toward the basal septum once THV is implanted, potentially obstructing the LVOT. The risk is higher for taller or pericardial valves, compared with shorter valves or porcine bioprostheses and long anterior leaflets (>25 mm) in patients with prior surgical repairs. Anatomic assessment

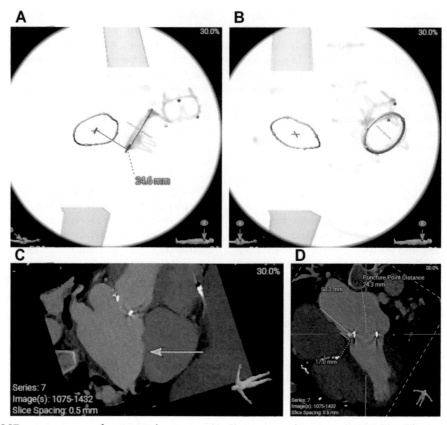

Fig. 2. CCT measurements of transseptal puncture. (*A*, *B*): Angiographic views. (*C*) Double oblique 4-chamber view. The yellow arrow denotes and optimal transseptal access location. (*D*) Transseptal puncture height 4-chamber view.

of the neo-LVOT on CCT is essential to help mitigate risk of LVOTO, and researchers have suggested that measurement during the phase of peak systolic flow may provide the most physiologic prediction of LVOTO (Fig. 4).[26] The CCT is instrumental because it allows simulated implantation of a virtual THV and subsequent calculation of the residual neo-LVOT and in cases of MViR, skirt neo-LVOT. Although the degree of residual neo-LVOT, which is acceptable, remains unclear, having a predicted neo-LVOT area less than 200 mm^2 is a significant risk factor for LVOTO, and a neo-LVOT area of less than 170 mm^2 predicts LVOTO with 96.2% sensitivity and 92.3% specificity.[25] Other risk factors for the development of LVOTO include the presence of

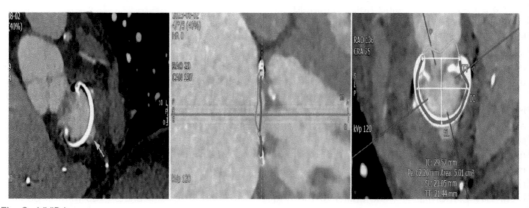

Fig. 3. MViR images.

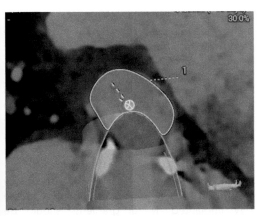

Fig. 4. Neo-LVOT measurement using CCT.

a bulky septum (>15 mm thickness), an acute aorto-mitral angle (<110°), an elongated anterior mitral leaflet (>25 mm), the presence of a small left ventricle cavity size (end-diastolic diameter <48 mm), left ventricular hypertrophy (LV mass index >105 g/m^2), or preserved ejection fraction.[19]

When a patient's assessment poses LVOTO risk, several strategies exist to help mitigate this risk. These include alcohol septal ablation (ASA), radiofrequency ablation, intentional leaflet laceration laceration of the anterior mitral valve leaflet to prevent outflow obstruction (LAMPOON), and more recently percutaneous myotomy Septal Scroring Along the Midline Endocardium (SESAME).[27] ASA is a well-established technique that eliminates the exaggerated septal bulge causing LVOTO, and increasing the neo-LVOT surface area by a median of 111.2 mm^2 (interquartile range: 71.4–193.1 mm^2).[28] Limitations of ASA, however, include the lack of septal perforators supplying salient myocardial tissue, thin septal myocardium and risk for ventricular septal defect formation, and induction of heart block.[27] A repeat CT is required after 4 to 8 weeks to reassess the neo-LVOT and TMVR candidacy. Alternatively, LAMPOON is an effective, although technically challenging procedure, which entails the use of catheter electrosurgery to lacerate the anterior leaflet and provide immediate neo-LVOT modification while sparing the myocardium.[27,29] Finally, radiofrequency ablation of the septum is a newer technique that is used much less frequently, and data surrounding its use remain limited.[27] Percutaneous myotomy is a new procedure still early its development that can be used to perform a controlled laceration of the basal septum and increase the LVOT area.[30]

Deciding on the best approach depends on several factors related to the patient's anatomy.

In brief, when both the frame and skirt neo-LVOT are less than 200 mm^2, the thickness of the interventricular septum should be assessed to determine whether the anatomy is suitable for ASA (ie, diastolic septal thickness ≥10 mm).[27] If ASA is not feasible or the neo-left ventricular outflow tract (neoLVOT) is still less than 200 mm^2 despite ASA on repeat CT 4 weeks later, then radiofrequency ablation may be indicated. In patients with a frame neoLVOT of less than 200 mm but a skirt neoLVOT greater than 200 mm^2, LAMPOON is the procedure of choice if the patient is a suitable candidate.[27] Factors that increase the success of LAMPOON include the following: (1) not having calcification in the central portion of the anterior leaflet to facilitate electrocautery laceration and (2) having sufficient anterior annular anchoring that can anchor the transcatheter valve once the anterior leaflet is lacerated.[27]

MANAGING POSTTRANSCATHETER MITRAL VALVE REPLACEMENT COMPLICATIONS

Left Ventricular Outflow Tract Obstruction

Although efforts should be made to preemptively mitigate the risk of LVOTO in high-risk patients as discussed earlier, LVOTO remains an inevitable complication in approximately 0.7% to 2.2% and 5% to 6% of patients undergoing MViV and MViR, respectively.[17,21] The development of LVOTO is associated with poor outcomes and increased risk of mortality.[27] In hemodynamically stable patients, medical management remains first-line therapy. Since both ventricular size and hypercontractility contribute to LVOTO, maintaining adequate volume status, using beta-blockers, avoiding inotropes, and using vasoconstrictors to increase afterload are important considerations for treatment in an acute situation.[31] In the case of hemodynamic instability, insertion of an Impella (Abiomed, Danvers, MA) is often done first. ASA or tip-to-base LAMPOON can then be attempted to relieve the obstruction. If not successful or feasible, then surgical revision would be required.[31]

Paravalvular Leak

PVL is a complication of TMVR, more commonly seen after MViR, which may present with symptoms of heart failure and, in some instances, may precipitate hemolytic anemia. In a prior analysis of 69 patients undergoing TMVR, PVL occurred in 3% of patients after MViV compared with 29% of patients MViR.[32] It could be due to geographic miss, ring dehiscence, or implantation of a THV into a rigid ring that does not provide adequate seal. Some operators have suggested that lengthening the THV landing zone by suturing additional graft material to extend the external skirt may improve annular sealing. Preliminary data have found that this may be an effective strategy for mitigating the incidence PVL without increasing complication risk.[33] Based on registry data from 40 European and American Centers, analysis of data from patients undergoing MViV (n = 322) and MViR (n = 141) found that PVL closure was required in 2.2% and 7.8% of cases, respectively.[34] Percutaneous PVL closure is sometimes performed via off-label use of septal or ductal occluder and vascular plug devices.[12]

Valve Embolization and Cardiac Perforation

Valve embolization is a rare but serious complication that occurs more frequently following MViR (2.4%) compared with MViV (0.1%).[35] The anchoring force of the THV is a result of the friction between the frame of the transcatheter prosthetic mitral valve and the surrounding tissue. Optimal deployment of the THV is necessary for generating this friction. When the THV is deployed too atrially, for instance, device stability may be compromised thus increasing the risk of embolization. Cardiac perforation is another rare but detrimental complication occurring in 1.9% to 2.4% of cases.[35] Emergency surgery is necessary to manage both conditions and associated with poor survival.

Anticoagulation Posttranscatheter Mitral Valve Replacement

Balancing the benefits of antithrombotic agents after TMVR with the risk of bleeding is another challenge that has yet to be thoroughly investigated. Although anticoagulation recommendations following mechanical or bioprosthetic SMVR exist, no specific recommendations are made for anticoagulation after TMVR.[36,37] Current anticoagulation strategies in TMVR are based on clinical experience and surgical literature.[32] Data on antithrombotic therapy are available on 411 of the 521 patients from the TMVR registry. Among these, 72% of patients were discharged on anticoagulation while 28% received antiplatelet therapy alone. At 1 year follow-up, the cumulative incidence of thrombosis was lower among those who received anticoagulation compared with those who did not (6.6% vs 1.6%; P = .019).[34] Another single-center study of 88 patients who underwent TMVR found that prosthetic valve thrombosis developed in 3% (2/67) of patients who were discharged on anticoagulation, compared with 28.6% (4/14) of patients

who were not.[32] Finally, another study of 1529 patients who underwent MViV, 81% of whom were anticoagulated, found that the incidence of valve thrombosis was 0.5% at 1 year follow-up.[17] Considered together, the evidence supports at least the short-term use of anticoagulation following TMVR, although further robust research is needed to explore the optimal type and duration of anticoagulation.

Postprocedural Gradients

Typical valve gradients post-TMVR are usually elevated (5–8 mm Hg) and are related to the THV implanted. Mitral gradients should be tracked immediately after THV implantation, and increases should prompt an investigation with either TEE or CCT to check for thrombus. In a TVT registry, patients receiving 23 mm Sapien 3 MViV were found to have 9.4 mm Hg gradients post-MViV. These elevated gradients were associated with higher rates of mortality at 1 year, and there are concerns about implanting 23 mm Sapien 3 valves with possible patient prosthesis mismatch afterward.[17] As for the concept intentional balloon fracture of surgical mitral valve for the purposes of implanting larger valves, it has been implemented but prospective data are still lacking.[38]

SUMMARY

Redo SMVR is associated with much higher risks than primary SMVR.[3,5] This has led to the emerging use of TMVR as an alternative to surgery, particularly in high-risk patients. Studies thus far have found that patients who undergo postsurgical TMVR have better outcomes and lower complication rates compared with those who undergo redo SMVR.[8,10,11] Postsurgical TMVR is certainly a promising option for degenerated bioprosthetic valves or annuloplasty rings; however, data thus far are limited to cohort and registry analyses. Further research is required to improve outcomes. Large trials are needed to evaluate the various aspects of procedural planning, procedural technique, and post-TMVR care.

CLINICS CARE POINTS

- Anatomic screeing using CT analysis for LVOT obstruction is key in the success in TMVR.
- TMVR requires a diverse skill set that includes transseptal access, alcohol septal ablation,

paravalvular leak repair, and familiarity with electrosurgical techniques such as LAMPOON.

- Transcatheter mitral valve-in-valve is safe, efficaciuous and highly reproducible.
- Transcatheter mitral valve-in-ring is nuanced and carries a higher complication and mortality rate than mitral valve-in-valve.

DISCLOSURES

M.H. Eng is a clinical proctor for Edwards Lifesciences and Medtronic. He is on the speaker's panel for Liva-Nova. H.K. Fang is on the speaker's bureau for Abbott. He is a consultant for Atricure and Edwards Lifesciences. The other authors have no conflict of interest.

REFERENCES

1. Coffey S, Roberts-Thomson R, Brown A, et al. Global epidemiology of valvular heart disease. Nat Rev Cardiol 2021;18(12):853–64.
2. Goldstone AB, Chiu P, Baiocchi M, et al. Mechanical or Biologic Prostheses for Aortic-Valve and Mitral-Valve Replacement. N Engl J Med 2017; 377(19):1847–57.
3. Bourguignon T, Bouquiaux-Stablo AL, Loardi C, et al. Very late outcomes for mitral valve replacement with the Carpentier-Edwards pericardial bioprosthesis: 25-year follow-up of 450 implantations. J Thorac Cardiovasc Surg 2014;148(5):2004–11.e1.
4. Kaneko T, Aranki S, Javed Q, et al. Mechanical versus bioprosthetic mitral valve replacement in patients <65 years old. J Thorac Cardiovasc Surg 2014;147(1):117–26.
5. Maganti M, Rao V, Armstrong S, et al. Redo valvular surgery in elderly patients. Ann Thorac Surg 2009; 87(2):521–5.
6. McCarthy KP, Ring L, Rana BS. Anatomy of the mitral valve: understanding the mitral valve complex in mitral regurgitation. Eur J Echocardiogr 2010;11(10):i3–9.
7. von Ballmoos MCW, Kalra A, Reardon MJ. Complexities of transcatheter mitral valve replacement (TMVR) and why it is not transcatheter aortic valve replacement (TAVR). Ann Cardiothorac Surg 2018; 7(6):724–30.
8. Zhou J, Li Y, Chen Z, et al. Transcatheter mitral valve replacement versus redo surgery for mitral prosthesis failure: A systematic review and meta-analysis. Front Cardiovasc Med 2023;9. https://doi.org/10.3389/FCVM.2022.1058576.
9. Goel K. Contemporary outcomes of transseptal mitral valve in valve in the United States, [oral presentation]. Phoenix AZ: Presented at TVT; 2023.
10. Khan MZ, Zahid S, Khan MU, et al. Redo Surgical Mitral Valve Replacement Versus Transcatheter Mitral Valve in Valve From the National Inpatient Sample. J Am Heart Assoc 2021;10(17).
11. Ismayl M, Abbasi MA, Mostafa MR, et al. Meta-Analysis Comparing Valve-in-Valve Transcatheter Mitral Valve Replacement Versus Redo Surgical Mitral Valve Replacement in Degenerated Bioprosthetic Mitral Valve. Am J Cardiol 2023;189: 98–107.
12. Garcia-Sayan E, Chen T, Khalique OK. Multimodality Cardiac Imaging for Procedural Planning and Guidance of Transcatheter Mitral Valve Replacement and Mitral Paravalvular Leak Closure. Front Cardiovasc Med 2021;8. https://doi.org/10.3389/FCVM.2021.582925.
13. Alperi A, Granada JF, Bernier M, et al. Current Status and Future Prospects of Transcatheter Mitral Valve Replacement: JACC State-of-the-Art Review. J Am Coll Cardiol 2021;77(24):3058–78.
14. Urena M, Himbert D, Brochet E, et al. Transseptal Transcatheter Mitral Valve Replacement Using Balloon-Expandable Transcatheter Heart Valves: A Step-by-Step Approach. JACC Cardiovasc Interv 2017;10(19):1905–19.
15. Grover FL, Vemulapalli S, Carroll JD, et al. Annual Report of The Society of Thoracic Surgeons/American College of Cardiology Transcatheter Valve Therapy Registry. J Am Coll Cardiol 2017;69(10): 1215–30.
16. Elmariah S, Fearon WF, Inglessis I, et al. Transapical Transcatheter Aortic Valve Replacement Is Associated With Increased Cardiac Mortality in Patients With Left Ventricular Dysfunction: Insights From the PARTNER I Trial. JACC Cardiovasc Interv 2017;10(23):2414–22.
17. Whisenant B, Kapadia SR, Eleid MF, et al. One-Year Outcomes of Mitral Valve-in-Valve Using the SAPIEN 3 Transcatheter Heart Valve. JAMA Cardiol 2020;1–8.
18. Simonato M, Forrest JK, Dvir D. The Dos and Don'ts of Mitral Valve-in-Valve and Valve-in-Ring. Innovat Tech Tech CardioThorac Vasc Surg 2021; 16(5):402–8.
19. Barreiro-Perez M, Caneiro-Queija B, Puga L, et al. Imaging in Transcatheter Mitral Valve Replacement: State-of-Art Review. J Clin Med 2021;10(24).
20. Pirelli L, Hong E, Steffen R, et al. Mitral valve-in-valve and valve-in-ring: tips, tricks, and outcomes. Ann Cardiothorac Surg 2021;10(1):96–112.
21. Simonato M, Whisenant B, Ribeiro HB, et al. Transcatheter Mitral Valve Replacement After Surgical Repair or Replacement Comprehensive Midterm Evaluation of Valve-in-Valve and Valve-in-Ring Implantation From the VIVID Registry. Circulation 2021;143(2):104–16.
22. Eng MH, Abbas AE. Transcatheter Mitral Valve Replacement in Failed Bioprosthetic Surgical

Valves and Surgical Annuloplasty Rings. Curr Cardiol Rep 2022;24(10):1417–24.

23. Greenbaum AB, Lisko JC, Gleason PT, et al. Annular-to-Apical "Emory Angle" to Ensure Coaxial Mitral Implantation of the SAPIEN 3 Valve. Cardiovasc Interv 2020;13(20):2447–50.

24. Eng MH, Verma DR. Mitral valve-in-ring: Simply complicated. Cathet Cardiovasc Interv 2021;97(2): 359–60.

25. Yoon S-H, Bleiziffer S, Latib A, et al. Predictors of Left Ventricular Outflow Tract Obstruction After Transcatheter Mitral Valve Replacement. JACC Cardiovasc Interv 2019;12(2):182–93.

26. Kohli K, Wei ZA, Sadri V, et al. Dynamic nature of the LVOT following transcatheter mitral valve replacement with LAMPOON: new insights from post-procedure imaging. Eur Hear journal Cardiovasc Imaging 2022;23(5):650–62.

27. Eleid MF, Collins JD, Mahoney P, et al. Emerging Approaches to Management of Left Ventricular Outflow Obstruction Risk in Transcatheter Mitral Valve Replacement. JACC Cardiovasc Interv 2023; 16(8):885–95.

28. Wang DD, Guerrero M, Eng MH, et al. Alcohol Septal Ablation to Prevent Left Ventricular Outflow Tract Obstruction During Transcatheter Mitral Valve Replacement: First-in-Man Study. JACC Cardiovasc Interv 2019;12(13):1268–79.

29. Kargoli F, Pagnesi M, Rahgozar K, et al. Current Devices and Complications Related to Transcatheter Mitral Valve Replacement: The Bumpy Road to the Top. Front Cardiovasc Med 2021;8:639058.

30. Khan JM, Bruce CG, Greenbaum AB, et al. Transcatheter Myotomy to Relieve Left Ventricular Outflow Tract Obstruction: The Septal Scoring Along the Midline Endocardium Procedure in Animals. Circ Cardiovasc Interv 2022;15(6):E011686.

31. Asgar AW, Ducharme A, Messas N, et al. Left Ventricular Outflow Tract Obstruction Following Mitral Valve Replacement: Challenges for Transcatheter Mitral Valve Therapy. Struct Hear 2018;2(5):372–9.

32. Eng MH, Kargoli F, Wang DD, et al. Short- and mid-term outcomes in percutaneous mitral valve replacement using balloon expandable valves. Cathet Cardiovasc Interv 2021;98(6):1193–203. https://doi.org/10.1002/CCD.29783.

33. Greenbaum AB, Perdoncin E, Paone G, et al. Tableside Skirt Modification of the SAPIEN 3 Valve to Reduce Paravalvular Leak During Transcatheter Mitral Valve Replacement. JACC Cardiovasc Interv 2021;14(8):932–4.

34. Yoon SH, Whisenant BK, Bleiziffer S, et al. Outcomes of transcatheter mitral valve replacement for degenerated bioprostheses, failed annuloplasty rings, and mitral annular calcification. Eur Heart J 2019;40(5):441–51.

35. Guerrero M, Vemulapalli S, Xiang Q, et al. Thirty-Day Outcomes of Transcatheter Mitral Valve Replacement for Degenerated Mitral Bioprostheses (Valve-in-Valve), Failed Surgical Rings (Valve-in-Ring), and Native Valve With Severe Mitral Annular Calcification (Valve-in-Mitral Annular Calcification) i. Circ Cardiovasc Interv 2020;13(3).

36. Otto CM, Nishimura RA, Bonow RO, et al. ACC/AHA Guideline for the Management of Patients With Valvular Heart Disease: A Report of the American College of Cardiology/American Heart Association Joint Committee on Clinical Practice Guidelines. Circulation 2021;143(5):E72–227.

37. Pagnesi M, Moroni F, Beneduce A, et al. Thrombotic Risk and Antithrombotic Strategies After Transcatheter Mitral Valve Replacement. JACC Cardiovasc Interv 2019;12(23):2388–401.

38. Kaneko T, Piccirillo B, Golwala H, et al. Balloon Fracture of a Surgical Mitral Bioprosthesis during Valve-in-Valve Transcatheter Mitral Valve Replacement: First-in-Human Report. Circ Cardiovasc Interv 2018;11(1):1–2.

Left Ventricular Outflow Tract Modification for Transcatheter Mitral Valve Replacement

Hiroki A. Ueyama, MD, Vasilis C. Babaliaros, MD,
Adam B. Greenbaum, MD*

KEYWORDS

- Transcatheter mitral valve replacement • Left ventricular outflow tract obstruction • LAMPOON
- SESAME • Alcohol septal ablation • Radiofrequency ablation

KEY POINTS

- Left ventricular outflow tract obstruction (LVOT) is a known life-threatening complication of transcatheter mitral valve replacement.
- The assessment of LVOT obstruction risk relies on pre-procedural computed tomographic measurements of neo-LVOT and skirt neo-LVOT.
- Various techniques for modifying the LVOT have been described, categorized into leaflet modification and septal reduction approaches.
- The proposed algorithm offers an effective means of identifying patients at risk of LVOT obstruction and facilitates the appropriate selection of LVOT modification techniques.

INTRODUCTION

Transcatheter mitral valve replacement (TMVR) has emerged as a promising alternative to surgical mitral valve replacement, offered in various settings, including valve-in-valve, valve-in-ring, and valve-in-MAC (mitral annular calcification) TMVR using a transcatheter aortic valve system in the mitral position. Investigational devices, such as Sapien M3 valve (Edwards Lifesciences, Irvine, California, USA), Tendyne valve (Abbott Vascular, Chicago, Illinois, USA), Intrepid valve (Medtronic, Minneapolis, Minnesota, USA), and AltaValve (4CMedical, Maple Grove, Minnesota, USA), are also being explored. However, early experience with TMVR has highlighted a concerning complication—left ventricular outflow tract (LVOT) obstruction. This complication occurs in up to 7% of TMVR cases, with valve-in-MAC TMVR having a notably higher incidence (40%) compared with valve-in-ring (5%) and valve-in-valve (2%) procedures.[1] The development of

LVOT obstruction is associated with a high in-hospital mortality rate exceeding 50%.[2] Consequently, the perceived risk of LVOT obstruction has become a leading cause of screen failure in TMVR registries.[3,4] Studies have successfully identified parameters in computed tomography (CT) that can reliably predict the risk of LVOT obstruction following TMVR. Moreover, various techniques have been described to mitigate this risk. This review article aims to explore the indications, procedural steps, and outcomes associated with available LVOT modification techniques to prevent obstruction after TMVR.

MECHANISM OF LEFT VENTRICULAR OUTFLOW TRACT OBSTRUCTION AFTER TRANSCATHETER MITRAL VALVE REPLACEMENT

The LVOT in a native heart is defined as the region bounded by the intervalvular fibrosa of the aortomitral continuity and the basal

Division of Cardiology, Emory Structural Heart and Valve Center, Emory University Hospital Midtown, 550 Peachtree Street, Northeast, Atlanta, GA 30306, USA
* Corresponding author. 550 Peachtree Street, Northeast, Atlanta, GA 30306.
E-mail address: adam.b.greenbaum@emory.edu

Intervent Cardiol Clin 13 (2024) 217–225
https://doi.org/10.1016/j.iccl.2023.11.002
2211-7458/24/© 2023 Elsevier Inc. All rights reserved.

anteroseptal wall.[5] In contrast to surgical mitral valve replacement, where the native leaflets are removed, transcatheter heart valve implantation in the mitral position involves pinning the anterior mitral leaflet open with the newly implanted valve frame. As a result, the leaflet is deflected toward the basal septum, creating a covered cylinder that protrudes into the LVOT. This displacement causes a shift in the original LVOT and the formation of an elongated and narrower LVOT, referred to as the "neo-LVOT" (Fig. 1).[5,6] Consequently, this displacement and narrowing of the LVOT can potentially compromise the forward flow of blood.

RISK PREDICTION

Success in TMVR heavily relies on pre-procedural comprehensive multimodality imaging analysis, particularly an electrocardiography-gated, contrast-enhanced cardiac CT. This imaging approach enables critical evaluations such as assessing the landing zone, determining valve size, performing virtual valve implantation, and stratifying the risk of LVOT obstruction.

Virtual valve implantation is performed during the end-systolic phase when the aortic valve remains open. Among various parameters investigated for predicting LVOT obstruction after TMVR, the "neo-LVOT area" and "skirt neo-LVOT area" have been extensively studied.[7-13] The neo-LVOT area refers to the cross-sectional area between the septal bulge and the most ventricular edge of the virtual valve frame, whereas the skirt neo-LVOT area is defined as the area between the septal bulge and the edge of the valve skirt (see Fig. 1). Neo-LVOT measurements less than 170 to 189 mm^2 have been established as reliable predictors of LVOT obstruction following TMVR.[8,9,11] Skirt neo-LVOT is measured when the leaflet modification technique (LAMPOON: Laceration of the Anterior Mitral leaflet to Prevent Outflow ObtructioN) is being considered during TMVR with transcatheter valves with partially open cell designs. Leaflet modification creates a split in the native anterior mitral leaflet, allowing for blood flow through the implanted valve struts. However, all current transcatheter valves still have a built-in "skirt" to prevent paravalvular leak that is not affected by this leaflet modification. Therefore, after leaflet modification, the neo-LVOT shifts to the edge of the valve skirt, hence the skirt neo-LVOT. A skirt neo-LVOT area of less than 150 to 180 mm^2 has been proposed as a risk of developing LVOT obstruction despite anterior leaflet modification.[12,13] Cases with septal hypertrophy, which often coincides with MAC-related mitral valve disease, tend to have narrow neo-LVOT and skirt neo-LVOT areas, risking LVOT obstruction.

LEFT VENTRICULAR OUTFLOW TRACT MODIFICATION TECHNIQUES

To address the risk of LVOT obstruction after TMVR, various techniques for LVOT modification have been developed. These approaches can be classified into two categories based on the specific structure of the LVOT being targeted: (1) leaflet modification, focusing on the anterior mitral leaflet and (2) septal reduction, targeting the basal septal bulge (Table 1).

Leaflet Modification

Leaflet modification involves creating a split in the anterior mitral leaflet to prevent it from sealing the implanted valve frame and creating

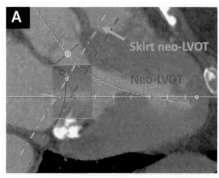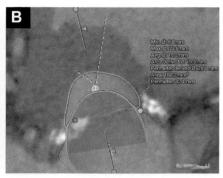

Fig. 1. Computed tomography modeling of virtual valve implantation and measurements of neo-LVOT and skirt neo-LVOT. (A) Virtual valve implanted in the native mitral annulus. Neo-LVOT is defined as cross-sectional area between most ventricular valve edge and septal bulge. Skirt neo-LVOT is defined as area between most ventricular edge of the skirt and septal bulge. (B) Cross-sectional area of skirt neo-LVOT measured with polygon function in 3mensio. LVOT, left ventricular outflow tract. (Image courtesy: Pie Medical Imaging B.V, Maastricht, The Netherlands.)

Table 1 Available left ventricular outflow tract modification techniques	
Leaflet Modification	**Septal Reduction**

• LAMPOON
  ○ Retrograde classic LAMPOON
  ○ Antegrade LAMPOON
  ○ Tip-to-base LAMPOON
  ○ Balloon-augmented LAMPOON
  ○ Rescue LAMPOON
	• Preemptive alcohol septal ablation
	• Preemptive radiofrequency ablation
	• SESAME

Abbreviations: LAMPOON, Laceration of the Anterior Mitral leaflet to Prevent Outflow ObtructioN; SESAME, Septal Scoring Along the Midline Endocardium.

an impermeable cylinder protruding into the LVOT. LAMPOON, first described in 2017,[14] has led to the development of several variants aimed at achieving more efficient and effective leaflet modification, each applied in different settings.

Retrograde classic Laceration of the Anterior Mitral leaflet to Prevent Outflow ObtructioN
Retrograde *classic* LAMPOON was the first iteration of this kind to use electrosurgery to lacerate the anterior mitral leaflet.

A guiding catheter is advanced retrograde into the LVOT, positioning it toward the base of the A2 mitral scallop. Another guiding catheter is also delivered retrograde through the LVOT, mitral valve, and into the left atrium. This guiding catheter is stabilized by creating a transeptal rail. A multiloop snare is delivered through this left atrial guiding catheter and positioned at the mitral coaptation surface. From the LVOT guiding catheter, a traversal guidewire is advanced from the left ventricular side of the leaflet, penetrating the A2 scallop with brief electrification, and then captured by the multiloop snare in the left atrium. A "flying V" configuration (a long steel guidewire with focally denuded insulation kinked at the midshaft to allow controlled radiofrequency laceration of the targeted tissue) is used to lacerate the anterior mitral leaflet, whereas both free end of the guiding catheter and the guidewire are pulled during electrification (Fig. 2).

The LAMPOON IDE trial studied 30 subjects at risk of LVOT obstruction following valve-in-MAC or valve-in-ring TMVR. The traversal and laceration were successful in all with no procedural death. Following TMVR, LVOT gradient

was acceptable (LVOT gradient < 50 mm Hg) in all cases.[15]

The splay created with retrograde *classic* LAMPOON aligns well with the LVOT by design. However, the limitation of this procedure lies in the technical difficulty of accurately placing the traversal guiding catheter to abut the base of the A2 scallop. It is important to note that this particular iteration of LAMPOON is not suitable for patients with a mechanical aortic valve, as it involves the delivery of two retrograde catheters through the aortic valve. Although seldomly still used in current practice, it may still have some utility in those with heavily calcified anterior leaflets.

Antegrade Laceration of the Anterior Mitral leaflet to Prevent Outflow ObtructioN
To overcome the limitations of retrograde *classic* LAMPOON, the technique of antegrade LAMPOON was developed.

In this approach, two deflectable sheaths are delivered through single transeptal puncture. One sheath is used to advance a balloon wedge end-hole catheter through the mitral orifice and out of the aortic valve. A guidewire advanced through this catheter is snared in the aorta, creating a rail. The balloon wedge end-hole catheter is then replaced with a guiding catheter, which is used to position a multiloop snare in the LVOT. Through the second transeptal deflectable sheath, another guiding catheter is advanced to abut the base of the A2 scallop from the atrial surface. A traversal guidewire is subsequently advanced penetrating the leaflet from the left atrium side of the leaflet and snared on the left ventricular side in the LVOT. A "flying V" configuration is used to lacerate the anterior mitral leaflet while simultaneously pulling both ends of the transeptal guiding catheter system (Fig. 3).

Antegrade LAMPOON has been described in a case series involving eight patients at risk of LVOT obstruction, and it was observed to have significantly shorter procedure times compared with the retrograde technique (39 ± 9 minutes vs 65 ± 35 minutes). The procedure was successful in all cases, with no instances of an increase in LVOT gradient greater than 10 mm Hg following TMVR.[16]

Antegrade LAMPOON has now become the standard approach due to its effectiveness, reproducibility, and simplified technique.[16] It is worth noting that this technique carries the risk of creating an eccentric laceration, which can be mitigated by accurately pivoting the two steerable sheaths.

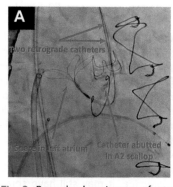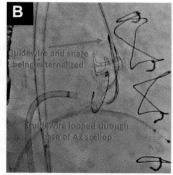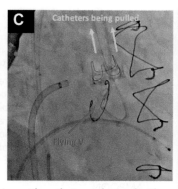

Fig. 2. Procedural angiogram of retrograde *classic* LAMPOON. (*A*) Two retrograde catheters advanced with one positioned abutting the A2 scallop and the other delivering a snare in the left atrium. (*B*) Guidewire ensnared and externalized. (*C*) Catheters pulled while applying electrosurgery at the flying V. LAMPOON, Laceration of the Anterior Mitral leaflet to Prevent Outflow ObtructioN.

Tip-to-base Laceration of the Anterior Mitral leaflet to Prevent Outflow ObtructioN

In a specific subset of patients with prior annuloplasty rings or bioprosthetic valve sewing rings protecting the aorto-mitral curtain, a simplified technique of tip-to-base LAMPOON can be performed. This approach obviates the need to traverse the A2 scallop at the base.

The tip-to-base LAMPOON technique involves delivering a steerable sheath to the left atrium through a transeptal approach. A balloon wedge end-hole catheter is then advanced through the mitral orifice and out of the aortic valve. A guidewire is passed through this catheter and subsequently snared, creating a venoarterial rail. Using this rail, the "flying V" configuration is advanced at the tip of the anterior mitral leaflet, and laceration is performed from the tip to the base (**Fig. 4**).

Tip-to-base LAMPOON has been reported in 21 patients with annuloplasty rings or valve prostheses protecting the aorto-mitral curtain. In all cases, the leaflet laceration was successful, and no instances of LVOT obstruction occurred following TMVR.[17]

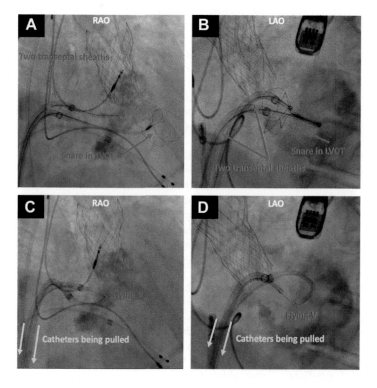

Fig. 3. Procedural angiogram of antegrade LAMPOON. (*A*, *B*) Two transeptal catheters advanced with one positioned abutting the A2 scallop and the other delivering a snare in the LVOT (*A*: RAO, *B*: LAO). (*C*, *D*) Catheters pulled while applying electrosurgery at the flying V (*C*: RAO, *D*: LAO). LAMPOON, Laceration of the Anterior Mitral leaflet to Prevent Outflow ObtructioN; LAO, left anterior oblique; LVOT, left ventricular outflow tract; RAO, right anterior oblique.

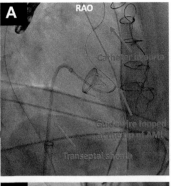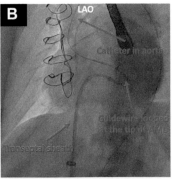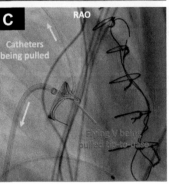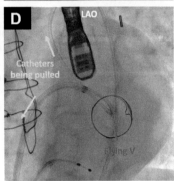

Fig. 4. Procedural angiogram of tip-to-base LAMPOON. (*A, B*) Guidewire forming a loop at the tip of anterior mitral leaflet (*A*: RAO, *B*: LAO). (*C, D*) Catheters pulled while applying electrosurgery at the flying V (*C*: RAO, *D*: LAO). AML, anterior mitral leaflet; LAMPOON, Laceration of the Anterior Mitral leaflet to Prevent Outflow ObstructioN; LAO, left anterior oblique; RAO, right anterior oblique.

It is important to note that this approach should only be used in patients who have sufficient protection of the aorto-mitral curtain, either through a surgical ring or a valve.

Balloon-augmented Laceration of the Anterior Mitral leaflet to Prevent Outflow ObstructioN

In cases where the anterior mitral leaflet is diffusely calcified and rigid, the conventional LAMPOON technique may not be sufficient to create an adequate splay and prevent LVOT obstruction. In such situations, balloon dilatation at the leaflet traversal site, performed before the electrosurgical laceration, has proven to effectively increase the splay. In a benchtop model, balloon-assisted laceration demonstrated significant improvements in leaflet tip splay (17% increase), maximum splay angle (30% increase), and splay area (23% increase).[18] In a series of patients with diffusely calcified leaflets who were determined to be at risk of inadequate leaflet splay with traditional LAMPOON, all patients underwent balloon-augmented LAMPOON successfully. Importantly, there were no cases of LVOT obstruction following TMVR in this patient cohort.[18]

Septal Reduction

Septal reduction strategies aim to address the opposing side of the structure that comprises the LVOT, specifically the bulging septum. Each strategy uses distinct mechanisms to decrease the extent of septal bulging, thereby augmenting the neo-LVOT. These procedures are considered when there is a persistent risk of LVOT obstruction despite LAMPOON.

Preemptive alcohol septal ablation

First described as an alternative to surgical myectomy for hypertrophic cardiomyopathy population with LVOT obstruction despite optimal medical therapy, alcohol septal ablation was then carried out as a bailout strategy in patients who developed LVOT obstruction after TMVR.[19] Subsequently, it has been studied as a preemptive strategy to prevent LVOT obstruction following TMVR.[20,21]

After confirming the septal perforator artery that supplies the basal anterior septum, an over-the-wire balloon is inserted and advanced. The balloon is then inflated to occlude and isolate the target artery from other arteries supplying non-targeted territories. Adequate positioning is assessed through selective angiography and echocardiographic contrast injection. Subsequently, a small volume of alcohol (usually 0.5–2.0 mL in preemptive cases for TMVR) is injected to intentionally induce an infarct in the respective area, thereby reducing septal thickness (Fig. 5).

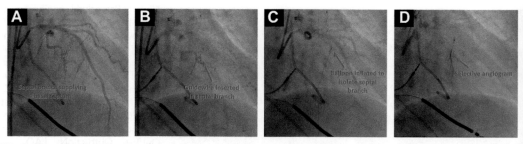

Fig. 5. Procedural angiogram of alcohol septal ablation. (A) Septal branch supplying basal septum identified. (B) Guidewire inserted in the septal branch. (C) Over-the-wire balloon inflated to isolate the septal branch. (D) Selective angiogram performed to confirm septal branch isolation.

In a prospective series comprising 30 patients who underwent preemptive alcohol septal ablation, the median augmentation in neo-LVOT was +111.2 m^2 (interquartile range: +71.4 to +193.1 mm^2). Pacemaker implantation occurred in 16.7%, and 30-day mortality was 10%.[20] In a separate series involving 22 patients, the average increase in neo-LVOT was 135 ± 89 mm^2. Of note, the pacemaker implantation rate in this series was 35%.[21]

Preemptive alcohol septal ablation holds appeal due to its relatively straightforward technique, which is familiar to interventional cardiologists based on experience with its use in hypertrophic cardiomyopathy. However, it necessitates the presence of an anatomically suitable septal perforator artery that supplies the basal septum. The notable incidence of pacemaker implantation should be acknowledged and factored into the informed decision-making process.

Preemptive radiofrequency ablation
Another septal reduction therapy built on the experience in hypertrophic cardiomyopathy[22] and used as a preemptive strategy in preventing LVOT obstruction following TMVR is the radiofrequency ablation.

This technique has thus far been documented only in a limited case series.[23,24] In one series involving four patients, a transseptal approach was used to guide the advancement of an externally irrigated ablation catheter to the septal bulge. Ablation was carried out until significant lesion formation was observed on intracardiac echocardiography, accompanied by the disappearance of electrograms at the target site.[23] The reported increase in neo-LVOT ranged from 7.6 to 110.3 mm^2, and skirt neo-LVOT ranged from 41.0 to 85.7 mm^2. All patients required pacemaker implantation, and despite successful ablation, three out of the four individuals remained at risk of developing LVOT obstruction. Similarly, in another series of five patients undergoing bipolar ablation of the basal septum, from both the left ventricular and right ventricular sides, the results showed a median increase in neo-LVOT of only 30 mm^2 (interquartile range: 0–60) and skirt neo-LVOT of 29 mm^2 (interquartile range: 10–53), with all patients requiring pacemaker implantation.[24]

Septal Scoring Along the Midline Endocardium
In order to address the limitations of existing septal reduction therapies, a transcatheter myotomy technique has been developed, aiming to replicate the initial surgical approach to hypertrophic obstructive cardiomyopathy. This technique involves creating a longitudinal splay along the septal bulge, with the goal of reducing septal encroachment and alleviating LVOT obstruction. The feasibility of this approach, known as the Septal Scoring Along the Midline Endocardium (SESAME) procedure, has been evaluated in animal studies, and the initial results from its first application in humans have been reported.[25,26]

Under fluoroscopy and transesophageal echocardiography guidance, a retrograde guiding catheter is used to engage the interventricular septum. A stiff guidewire with tip cutoff nested within a microcatheter is embedded in the ventricular septum. The guidewire is advanced along a predetermined path within the myocardium until it reenters the left ventricular cavity. Subsequently, the guidewire is ensnared and a "flying V" is introduced to the distal border of the septum. The "flying V" is then energized and pulled, resulting in the creation of a splay in the myocardium extending from the mid-septum to the basal septum (Fig. 6).

A first-in-human experience of SESAME to prevent LVOT obstruction following TMVR has been reported, demonstrating successful

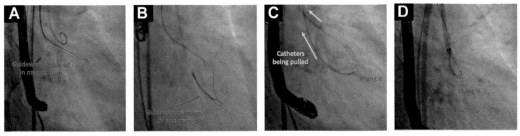

Fig. 6. Procedural angiogram of SESAME. (*A*) Guidewire advanced in the myocardium. (*B*) Guidewire reentered the left ventricle and ensnared. (*C*) Catheters pulled while applying electrosurgery at the flying V. (*D*) Flying V further pulled. LV, left ventricle; SESAME, Septal Scoring Along the Midline Endocardium.

augmentation of LVOT measurements and achievement of TMVR without the emergence of LVOT gradient.[25] A noteworthy characteristic of SESAME is its distinctive engagement of the septum between the native right–left commissure and the nadir of the right coronary sinus, thus avoiding interference with conduction system. A case series conducted at a single center is currently underway, showing promising results thus far.

ALGORITHM

To facilitate a streamlined and systematic assessment of LVOT obstruction risk and the selection of LVOT modification techniques before TMVR, we have developed a straightforward algorithm (Fig. 7). Briefly, the algorithm involves the following steps.

1. Measure neo-LVOT. Considering a safety margin from previous reports, neo-LVOT < 200 mm^2 is considered at risk of LVOT obstruction.
2. If the measured skirt neo-LVOT ≥ 180 mm^2, LAMPOON alone should be sufficient to mitigate the risk of LVOT obstruction.
3. If the measured skirt neo-LVOT is < 180 mm^2, preemptive septal reduction therapy should be performed to reduce the risk of LVOT obstruction despite LAMPOON.
4. If the skirt neo-LVOT remains < 180 mm^2 despite septal reduction therapy, the patient remains at risk of LVOT obstruction, and alternative septal reduction techniques or a surgical approach should be reconsidered if feasible.
5. If the skirt neo-LVOT ≥ 180 mm^2 and the neo-LVOT ≥ 200 mm^2, the patient is now at low

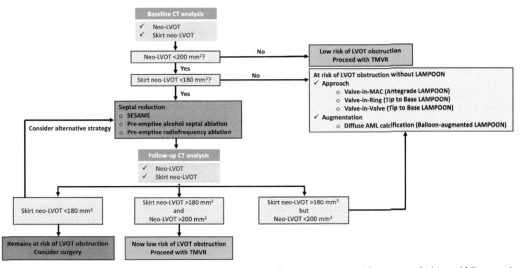

Fig. 7. Algorithm on assessing LVOT obstruction risk and selecting LVOT modification technique. AML, anterior mitral leaflet; CT, computed tomography; LAMPOON, Laceration of the Anterior Mitral leaflet to Prevent Outflow ObtructioN; LVOT, left ventricular outflow tract; MAC, mitral annular calcification; SESAME, Septal Scoring Along the Midline Endocardium; TMVR, transcatheter mitral valve replacement. (Vasilis C. Babaliaros et al., The Art of SAPIEN 3 Transcatheter Mitral Valve Replacement in Valve-in-Ring and Valve-in-Mitral-Annular-Calcification Procedures, JACC: Cardiovascular Interventions, 14 (20), 2021, 2195-2214, https://doi.org/10.1016/j.jcin.2021.08.044.)

risk of developing LVOT obstruction and can proceed with TMVR without further adjunctive measures.

6. If the skirt neo-LVOT $\geq$ 180 mm^2, but the neo-LVOT < 200 mm^2, LAMPOON should be performed to facilitate TMVR.

SUMMARY

Early experiences with unfavorable outcomes have fostered a comprehensive comprehension of the interplay between TMVR and LVOT, subsequently driving the development of various techniques to mitigate the risk of LVOT obstruction. The key to successful TMVR lies in being adaptable in risk assessment and being equipped with a diverse array of LVOT modification techniques.

CLINICS CARE POINTS

- LVOT obstruction occurs in up to 7% of TMVR cases, with valve-in-MAC TMVR having notably higher incidence of 40%.

- Development of LVOT obstruction is associated with a high in-hospital mortality reaching up to 50%.

- neo-LVOT < 200mm2 and skirt neo-LVOT < 180 mm2 is considered high risk of LVOT obstruction following TMVR.

- LVOT modification techniques include LAMPOON, SESAME, alcohol septal ablation, and radiofrequency ablation.

DISCLOSURE

A.B. Greenbaum receives proctor honoraria from Edwards Lifesciences. A.B. Greenbaum and V.C. Babaliaros have equity interest in Transmural Systems.

REFERENCES

1. Yoon SH, Whisenant BK, Bleiziffer S, et al. Outcomes of transcatheter mitral valve replacement for degenerated bioprostheses, failed annuloplasty rings, and mitral annular calcification. Eur Heart J 2019;40(5):441–51.

2. Guerrero M, Urena M, Himbert D, et al. 1-year outcomes of transcatheter mitral valve replacement in patients with severe mitral annular calcification. J Am Coll Cardiol 2018;71(17):1841–53.

3. Guerrero M, Wang DD, Pursnani A, et al. Prospective evaluation of TMVR for failed surgical annuloplasty rings: MITRAL trial valve-in-ring arm 1-year

outcomes. JACC Cardiovasc Interv 26 2021;14(8): 846–58.

4. Guerrero M, Wang DD, Eleid MF, et al. Prospective study of TMVR using balloon-expandable aortic transcatheter valves in MAC: MITRAL trial 1-year outcomes. JACC Cardiovasc Interv 2021;14(8): 830–45.

5. Reid A, Zekry SB, Turaga M, et al. Neo-LVOT and Transcatheter Mitral Valve Replacement. JACC (J Am Coll Cardiol): Cardiovascular Imaging 2021; 14(4):854–66.

6. Blanke P, Naoum C, Webb J, et al. Multimodality imaging in the context of transcatheter mitral valve replacement: establishing consensus among modalities and disciplines. JACC (J Am Coll Cardiol): Cardiovascular Imaging 2015;8(10):1191–208.

7. Urena M, Himbert D, Brochet E, et al. Transseptal transcatheter mitral valve replacement using balloon-expandable transcatheter heart valves: a step-by-step approach. JACC Cardiovasc Interv 2017;10(19):1905–19.

8. Sabbagh AE, Al-Hijji M, Wang DD, et al. Predictors of left ventricular outflow tract obstruction after transcatheter mitral valve replacement in severe mitral annular calcification: an analysis of the transcatheter mitral valve replacement in mitral annular calcification global registry. Circulation: Cardiovascular Interventions 2021;14(10):e010854.

9. Yoon SH, Bleiziffer S, Latib A, et al. predictors of left ventricular outflow tract obstruction after transcatheter mitral valve replacement. JACC Cardiovasc Interv 2019;12(2):182–93.

10. Greenbaum AB, Condado JF, Eng M, et al. Long or redundant leaflet complicating transcatheter mitral valve replacement: Case vignettes that advocate for removal or reduction of the anterior mitral leaflet. Cathet Cardiovasc Interv 2018;92(3):627–32.

11. Wang DD, Eng MH, Greenbaum AB, et al. Validating a prediction modeling tool for left ventricular outflow tract (LVOT) obstruction after transcatheter mitral valve replacement (TMVR). Cathet Cardiovasc Interv 2018;92(2):379–87.

12. Khan JM, Rogers T, Babaliaros VC, et al. Predicting Left Ventricular Outflow Tract Obstruction Despite Anterior Mitral Leaflet Resection: The "Skirt Neo-LVOT". JACC Cardiovasc Imaging 2018;11(9):1356–9.

13. Kohli K, Wei ZA, Sadri V, et al. Dynamic nature of the LVOT following transcatheter mitral valve replacement with LAMPOON: new insights from post-procedure imaging. European Heart Journal - Cardiovascular Imaging 2021;23(5):650–62.

14. Babaliaros VC, Greenbaum AB, Khan JM, et al. Intentional Percutaneous Laceration of the Anterior Mitral Leaflet to Prevent Outflow Obstruction During Transcatheter Mitral Valve Replacement: First-in-Human Experience. JACC Cardiovasc Interv 2017;10(8):798–809.

15. Khan JM, Babaliaros VC, Greenbaum AB, et al. Anterior leaflet laceration to prevent ventricular outflow tract obstruction during transcatheter mitral valve replacement. J Am Coll Cardiol 2019; 73(20):2521–34.

16. Lisko JC, Greenbaum AB, Khan JM, et al. ante-grade intentional laceration of the anterior mitral leaflet to prevent left ventricular outflow tract obstruction: a simplified technique from bench to bedside. Circ Cardiovasc Interv 2020;13(6):e008903.

17. Lisko JC, Babaliaros VC, Khan JM, et al. Tip-to-Base LAMPOON for Transcatheter Mitral Valve Replacement With a Protected Mitral Annulus. JACC Cardiovasc Interv 2021;14(5):541–50.

18. Perdoncin E, Bruce CG, Babaliaros VC, et al. balloon-augmented leaflet modification with bio-prosthetic or native aortic scallop intentional lacer-ation to prevent iatrogenic coronary artery obstruction and laceration of the anterior mitral leaflet to prevent outflow obstruction: benchtop validation and first in-man experience. Circ Cardio-vasc Interv 2021;14(11):e011028.

19. Guerrero M, Wang DD, Himbert D, et al. Short-term results of alcohol septal ablation as a bail-out strat-egy to treat severe left ventricular outflow tract obstruction after transcatheter mitral valve replace-ment in patients with severe mitral annular calcifica-tion. Cathet Cardiovasc Interv 2017;90(7):1220–6.

20. Wang DD, Guerrero M, Eng MH, et al. Alcohol Septal Ablation to Prevent Left Ventricular Outflow Tract Obstruction During Transcatheter Mitral Valve Replacement: First-in-Man Study. JACC Car-diovasc Interv 2019;12(13):1268–79.

21. Elhadi M, Guerrero M, Collins JD, et al. Safety and Outcomes of Alcohol Septal Ablation Prior to Transcatheter Mitral Valve Replacement. Journal of the Society for Cardiovascular Angiography & In-terventions 2022;1(5). https://doi.org/10.1016/j.jscai.2022.100396.

22. Crossen K, Jones M, Erikson C. Radiofrequency septal reduction in symptomatic hypertrophic obstructive cardiomyopathy. Heart Rhythm 2016; 13(9):1885–90.

23. Killu AM, Collins JD, Eleid MF, et al. Preemptive septal radiofrequency ablation to prevent left ventricular outflow tract obstruction with trans-catheter mitral valve replacement: a case series. Circulation: Cardiovascular Interventions 2022; 15(10):e012228.

24. Hoskins MH, Lisko JC, Greenbaum AB, et al. Septal bipolar ablation to prevent left ventricular outflow tract obstruction after transcatheter mitral valve im-plantation. Circ Cardiovasc Interv 2023;e013333. https://doi.org/10.1161/circinterventions.123.013333.

25. Greenbaum AB, Khan JM, Bruce CG, et al. Trans-catheter myotomy to treat hypertrophic cardiomy-opathy and enable transcatheter mitral valve replacement: first-in-human report of septal scoring along the midline endocardium. Circ Cardi-ovasc Interv 2022;15(6):e012106.

26. Khan JM, Bruce CG, Greenbaum AB, et al. Transcath-eter myotomy to relieve left ventricular outflow tract obstruction: the septal scoring along the midline endocardium procedure in animals. Circulation: Car-diovascular Interventions 2022;15(6):e011686.

Orthotopic Transcatheter Mitral Valve Replacement

Marvin H. Eng, MD[a],*, Firas Zahr, MD[b]

KEYWORDS

- Orthotopic • Mitral valve • Left ventricular outflow tract obstruction
- Transcatheter mitral valve replacement

KEY POINTS

- Mitral annular variability, left ventricular size, and left ventricular outflow tract obstruction are significant constraints to transcatheter mitral valve replacement (TMVR).
- Rigorous analysis of 3-dimensional computed tomography with prosthesis modeling is required to successfully screen for TMVR.
- Clinical evaluation of patient characteristics such as ejection fraction, susceptibility to bleeding with anticoagulation, and optimization of heart failure therapy is a key part of patient selection for TMVR.
- Orthotopic TMVR requires a prosthesis with stable anchoring, adequate sealing, small footprint in the left ventricle, and long-term durability.

BACKGROUND

Mitral valve dysfunction is highly prevalent across elderly populations and increases with age.[1] As patients advance in age, their eligibility for surgery declines, prompting clinicians to consider transcatheter alternatives. It should be noted that a minority of patients with mitral regurgitation (MR) are treated and large populations are not offered surgical repair or replacement.[1]

Mitral pathology is diverse and is generalized into 2 broad categories: degenerative and functional. Degenerative, also commonly referred as primary, refers to malcoaptation as a result of structural leaflet abnormalities such as prolapse or flail due to chordal disruption. Functional regurgitation indicates that the leaflets themselves are structurally normal but malcoaptation results from cardiac remodeling causing any combination of annular dilation or leaflet tethering from ventricular dilation or dysfunction. Furthermore, patients can manifest combinations of both phenotypes along with a broad range of pathologies that may include simultaneous stenosis and regurgitation, leaflet or annular calcification, fibrosis or healed endocarditis, and leaflet perforations.

Mitral transcatheter edge-to-edge repair (TEER) is a percutaneous therapy based on the Alfieri principle of plicating the mitral valve at the location of malcoaptation and is currently approved for high-risk and inoperative degenerative and functional MR patients but bears limitations.[2,3] Patients with multiple jets, mitral annular or leaflet calcification, small mitral orifice area, commissural jets, large coaptation gaps, and baseline mitral stenosis can result in suboptimal results.[4,5] Moderate residual MR attenuates survival in patients undergoing TEER and there is a need to achieve less than moderate regurgitation.[6] Additionally, some TEER cases result in leaflet damage and poor tissue integrity may render TEER unusable.[7] Complementary tools for treatment of MR are needed given the limitations of mitral TEER.

Native Anatomy Relevant to Transcatheter Mitral Valve Replacement

The challenges of orthotopic transcatheter mitral valve replacement (TMVR) are largely related to

---

[a] Structural Heart Program, Division of Cardiology, University of Arizona, Banner University Medical Center, 755 East McDowell Road, Phoenix, AZ 85006, USA; [b] Division of Cardiovascular Medicine, Knight Cardiovascular Institute, Oregon Health & Science University, Portland, OR, USA

* Corresponding author.

E-mail address: marvin.eng@bannerhealth.com

the intricacies of mitral valve anatomy (Fig. 1).[8] Recall that the mitral valve is dynamic with a sub-valvular component. The valve is composed of a saddle-shaped, semi-rigid annulus that is D-shaped, as well as the anterior and posterior mitral valve leaflets. The leaflets are tethered to collagenous chordae tendineae arising from the papillary muscles to support the leaflets during systole. Furthermore, the anterior mitral leaflet is adjacent to the left ventricular (LV) outflow track (LVOT) and can interact with systolic flow if displaced anteriorly by a prothesis.[9] The combination of the asymmetric D-shape configuration, an annulus with limited rigidity, subvalvular apparatus, and outflow tract proximity makes orthotopic TMVR an anatomic challenge for prosthesis fixation, adequate sealing, and avoiding LVOT obstruction (LVOTO).

TRANSCATHETER MITRAL VALVE REPLACEMENT KEYS TO SUCCESS

At the time of this review, TMVR remains investigational in the US and TENDYNE is CE (Conformite Europeenne)–marked in Europe. Several features determine patient eligibility and success for TMVR: access; anatomic eligibility; patient selection; and durability.

Access
Transapical and transseptal access are currently the routes utilized for transcatheter heart valve (THV) delivery. The advantage to transapical access includes coaxial delivery of prosthesis and enhanced control over THV positioning for implantation. However, the transapical access is associated with high rates of bleeding and atrial fibrillation.[10,11] Meanwhile, transseptal access begins with venous and transseptal access; therefore, all of the maneuvering is performed in the left atrium and coaxial THV deployment can be difficult. When comparing the 2 access routes, the Society of Thoracic Surgeons (STS) and the American College of Cardiology Transcatheter Valve Therapy Registry of commercial balloon-expandable TMVR for valve-in-valve (ViV) procedures reported that transseptal access was associated with shorter lengths of hospital stay (2 vs 6 days, P<.001) and lower 1-year all-cause mortality (15.8% vs 21.7%, respectively, P = .03) relative to transapical access.[12] Early experience with the Intrepid (Medtronic, St. Paul, MN) valve noted 5 reoperations for transapical bleeding and an 18% procedural major bleeding.[13] It should be noted that early experience with mostly transapical first-generation TMVR reported an 11.2% rate of major bleeding which was associated with a 2.85-fold (confidence interval [CI] 1.6–4.9, P<.0001) increase in mortality.[14] Current experience of orthotopic TMVR showed trends toward lower rates of all-cause mortality with transseptal access. One caveat with transseptal access is size of delivery catheters tend to be large and access site bleeding must be respected.[15] For example, the current transfemoral Intrepid delivery sheath is 35-French (Fr) and requires a surgical cut-down.

Patient Selection
Appropriate patient selection for TMVR includes the typical clinical assessment with some unique facets. Usual predictors of survival such as age, chronic kidney disease, atherosclerotic burden, and lung function remain important considerations for long-term survival. Real-world observations of commercial TMVR for mitral ViV patients demonstrated significant survival differences stratified by STS-predicted mortality projections.[12]

Patients eligible for TMVR tend to have functional MR and LV systolic dysfunction.[16] As such,

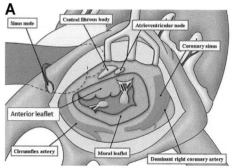
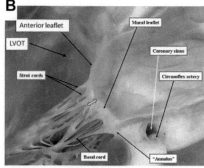

Fig. 1. Native mitral valve anatomy. (A) Cartoon depiction of native mitral anatomy and surrounding structures from the left atrial perspective. (B) Profile view of the native mitral valve. Note that the anterior leaflet borders the LVOT and anterior displacement narrows the LVOT. LVOT, left ventricular outflow tract. Double headed arrow is the mitral valve. (Adapted and reprinted from Van Mieghem N et al. J Am Coll Cardiol 2010;56:617-26 with permission from Elsevier.[8])

these patients require appropriate best practices for cardiomyopathy management prior to consideration of mitral valve therapies that may include medical optimization, resynchronization therapy, revascularization, and rhythm management.[3] Additionally, the low afterload state of the ventricle with MR disguises the true severity of LV function and the true function of the LV may not be appreciated until restoration of mitral competency as observed in the early TMVR experience where LV ejection fraction (LVEF) post-TMVR was significantly lower in follow-up.[13,17] Furthermore, the acute increase in ventricular afterload with a mitral valve replacement and concerns for afterload mismatch prompt clinicians to avoid severe dilated cardiomyopathies. Data regarding afterload mismatch in transcatheter mitral interventions are relatively scant but a recent analysis of LVEF decline post-mitral TEER found that patients with degenerative MR had significantly worse survival compared to patients with functional MR.[18]

A second critical issue with TMVR patient selection is suitability for anticoagulation. TMVR registries have shown valve thrombosis rates of 6% to 7%.[19,20] If not discharged on anticoagulation, valve thrombosis rates can climb to 29%.[19] Clearly, chronic anticoagulation is important for valve function and potentially durability. However, bleeding is a concern as a 2% to 4% rate of late major bleeding was observed in registries.[15,19] The duration of anticoagulation is yet to be determined and it is unclear if surgical guidelines for anticoagulation are applicable to mitral THVs.

Anatomic Eligibility
Mitral anatomy is highly variable and when looking at the reasons for patient exclusion from TMVR, 79% of patients were excluded due to anatomic variables.[10] These include: annular size, small LV size, leaflet morphology, mitral annular calcification (MAC) and LVOTO. Currently, investigational TMVR is limited in prosthesis sizes and depending on the fixation mechanism of the prosthesis, the range of TMVR treatment is limited according to the combination of matching prosthesis size and the rest of the LV anatomy for anatomic eligibility. MAC remains a challenging anatomic obstacle and early data for treating with balloon-expandable valves demonstrated high early mortality and morbidity rates.[21] A comprehensive review of orthotopic TMVR for MAC patients is beyond the scope of this article and deserves a dedicated review, and orthotopic

TMVR specifically for MAC will be discussed elsewhere in this issue.

LVOTO (Fig. 2) remains a significant rate limiting factor in performing TMVR with the current generation of investigational devices. Significant morbidity and mortality result from LVOTO and the use of 3-dimensional computed tomography (CT) is compulsory for all TMVR screening.[22,23] Based on observational registries, the inflection point for LVOTO appears to be greater than 170 to 190 mm^2.[22–25] It is unclear if this is prosthesis specific and neo-LVOT modeling is unique to each valve type. A more recent analysis suggests that since 95% of blood volume is ejected by 30% of the R-R interval, a cut-off of 150 mm^2 at 30% of the R-R would be sufficient for the Intrepid valve.[26] Since LVOTO is caused by anterior displacement of the anterior mitral leaflet toward the basal ventricular septum, anterior leaflet morphology plays a role in LVOTO.[27] Certain valves are designed to circumvent this LVOTO as much as possible such as the Alta valve, but LVOTO screening remains a critical issue in TMVR anatomic eligibility. Mitigation of LVOTO extends beyond the scope of this review and is covered elsewhere.

TRANSCATHETER MITRAL VALVE REPLACEMENT: TRANSCATHETER HEART VALVES IN DEVELOPMENT
Idealized Transcatheter Mitral Valve Replacement
Optimal safety and efficacy for TMVR is a complex challenge. Anatomically, an ideal TMVR would be able to accommodate a broad range of annular sizes, including large annular dimensions. The ventricular profile should be minimal to minimize the possibility for LVOTO. Sealing needs to be excellent to prevent paravalvular leak (PVL) and hemolysis as moderate or greater PVL is associated with ~2-fold increase in 1-year mortality.[28] Transfemoral, transseptal access has a more favorable safety profile but the delivery mechanism needs to articulate in a favorable way for coaxial prosthesis delivery and low profile enough to obviate surgical cutdown. Finally, the PVL and valve performance need to be durable with a short duration of oral anticoagulation for thromboprophylaxis. A registry of contemporary TMVR found that only 41% of patients screened passed for implantation with first-generation dedicated orthotopic TMVR devices.[16] None of the current investigational devices encompasses all of these characteristics and the authors will briefly discuss some contemporary investigational

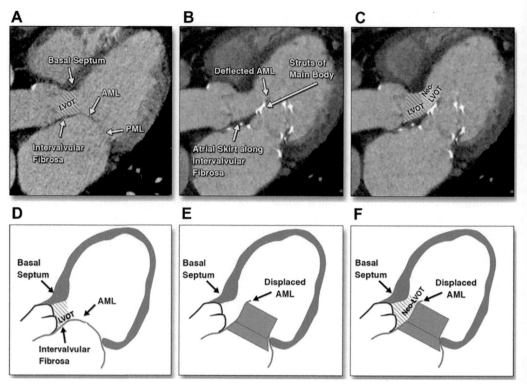

Fig. 2. Concept of the Neo-left ventricular outflow tract in transcatheter mitral valve replacement. (*Upper row*) End-systolic 3-chamber view on cardiac computed tomography. (*Lower row*) Schematic drawing. Before TMVR, the LVOT is confined by the basal septum, the intervalvular fibrosa, and basal portion of the AML (*A and D*). The TMVR device deflects the AML "septally," thereby elongating the outflow tract toward the left ventricle (*B and E*). This elongation is referred to as neo-LVOT, confined by the basal septum and the septally deflected AML (*C and F*). AML, anterior mitral valve leaflet; LVOT, left ventricular outflow tract; TMVR, transcatheter mitral valve replacement. (*Reprinted from* Blanke P et al. JACC: Cardiovascular Imaging; 2017:10 (4): 482-5 with permission from Elsevier.[9])

devices in development at this time. While the valves discussed in this review are not exhaustive, they illustrate the THV's current clinical development and the gamut of innovation for TMVR (Table 1).

Sapien M3 (Edwards Lifesciences, Irvine, CA, USA)

The Sapien M3 (see Fig. 3A–C) is composed a sub-annular dock that encircles the entire leaflet and subvalvular apparatus to enable implantation of a balloon-expandable valve.[29] A 29-mm Sapien valve has been modified to have the entire cobalt-chromium frame to be covered by graft material to minimize PVL. The sub-annular dock is deployed from the left atrium via transseptal puncture and the encircling process begins at the medial commissure with the ultimate goal of 3 encircling turns and deployment of an atrial turn in the left atrium. The dock has a hydrophilic coat to improve ease of implantation that is then removed. The dock passes through the medial commissure from

the ventricle to the left atrium and a PVL guard is embedded to mitigate leaking. The balloon-expandable valve is deployed with rapid pacing within the dock.

The most up-to-date data regarding M3 outcomes includes data from the early feasibility study. Acute technical success was 88.6% and 1-month follow-up observed 2.9% mortality with a 12.1% rate of ≥moderate MR.[30]

Intrepid (Medtronic)

The Intrepid valve (see Fig. 3D–F) is a self-expanding, nitinol prosthesis that anchors via radial force and oversizing with the assistance of multiple small frictional cleats.[13] The prosthesis has a flared ventricular end, narrower annular contact, and a wide-based atrial brim. There is an outer stent for anchoring and a smaller stent nested within that houses a bovine pericardial valve. It has both transapical and transseptal approaches. Depending on the approach, a straight or curved sheath positions the valve in the left atrium and the atrial brim

Table 1
Investigational transcatheter mitral valve replacement

Device	Design	Fixation	Access	Sheath	Annulus Target
Sapien M3 (Edwards Lifesciences, Irvine, CA, USA) (Fig. 3A–C)	Subannular nitinol dock Balloon-expandable bovine valve	Dock and valve trap the mitral leaflets	Transseptal	28-Fr	Up to 50 mm
Intrepid (Medtronic, St. Paul, MN, USA) (Fig. 3D–F)	Self-expanding double-frame bovine valve	Radial force and anchoring cleats	Transapical or transseptal	35-Fr	28–52 mm
Tendyne (Abbott Structural, Santa Clara, CA, USA) (Fig. 3G–I)	Self-expanding nitinol porcine valve with double-frame design	Apical tether	Transapical	38-Fr	101–143 mm (perimeter)
Cephea (Abbott Structural, Santa Clara, CA, USA) (Fig. 4A–C)	Self-expanding bovine valve double-disc design	Radial force and axial compression	Transseptal	36-Fr	25–46 mm
Highlife (Highlife SAS, Irvine, CA, USA) (Fig. 4D–F)	Self-expanding bovine valve with a subannular dock	Dock and valve trap leaflets	Transapical or Transseptal + transarterial	30-Fr	30–53 mm
Cardiovalve (Venus Medtech, Hangzhou, CN) (Fig. 4G–I)	Self-expanding nitinol frame, bovine valve	Annular anchoring and atrial flanges	Transseptal	32-Fr	36–53 mm
Alta Valve (4C Medical, Maple Grove, MN, USA) (Fig. 4K, L)	Self-expanding nitinol frame with minimal ventricular profile	Left atrial oversizing	Transseptal or transapical	29-Fr	29–51 mm

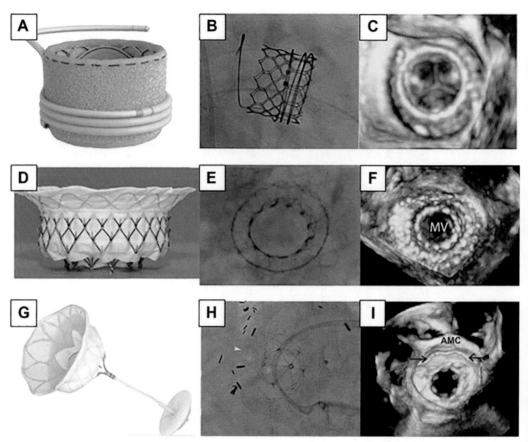

Fig. 3. Selected transcatheter mitral valve prostheses. (*A–C*) Sapien M3 docking system. (*A*) Ex-vivo prosthesis, (*B*) fluoroscopic image of the valve, (*C*) 3-dimensional transesophageal echocardiography (3D-TEE) imaging from the left atrial perspective. (*D–F*) Intrepid valve. (*D*) Ex-vivo prosthesis, (*E*) fluoroscopic image of the valve, (*F*) 3D-TEE image from the left atrium. (*G–I*) Tendyne valve. (*G*) Ex-vivo prosthesis, (*H*) fluoroscopic image of the valve, *Arrowhead* indicates the atrial flange of the Tendyne valve. (*I*) 3D-TEE image from the left atrium. (*Data from* ([*A-C*] John G. Webb et al. Percutaneous Transcatheter Mitral Valve Replacement: First-in-Human Experience With a New Transseptal System,Journal of the American College of Cardiology, 73 (11), 2019, 1239-1246, https://doi.org/ 10.1016/j.jacc.2018.12.065.); and ([*D-F*] John Webb et al. Transcatheter Mitral Valve Replacement With the Transseptal EVOQUE System, JACC: Cardiovascular Interventions, 13 (20), 2020, 2418-2426, https://doi.org/10.1016/ j.jcin.2020.06.040.); and ([*G, H*] Alberto Alperi et al., Early Experience With a Novel Transfemoral Mitral Valve Implantation System in Complex Degenerative Mitral Regurgitation, JACC: Cardiovascular Interventions, 13 (20), 2020, 2427-2437, https://doi.org/10.1016/j.jcin.2020.08.006.))[34]

makes initial contact. Subsequently, the valve deploys from atrial side to ventricular side using a hydraulic system with simultaneous rapid pacing.

Results of the early transapical experience reported a 50-patient cohort with a 96% intentional-to-treat success rate and 5 reoperations for rebleeding. The 30-day and 1-year survival rates were 86% and 76.5%, respectively. Follow-up echocardiograms revealed mild MR in 26% of patients with a mix of paravalvular and valvular regurgitation.[13]

Early feasibility of the transseptal Intrepid system recently reported a 94% technical success rate with a 30-day and 1-year survival of 100% and 93.3% survival rate, respectively.[31] The 35-Fr delivery system contributes to a 24.2% rate of vascular complications. One-year assessment found a 4% rate of mild MR and a 92% rate of New York Heart Association (NYHA) I to II symptoms. Patient screening remains a challenge with Intrepid due to both constraints with respect to projected LVOTO and vascular access but a lower profile delivery system may improve success.

Tendyne (Abbott Structural, Santa Clara, CA, USA)

The Tendyne THV (see **Fig. 3**G–I) is a transapically implanted D-shaped, nitinol prosthesis

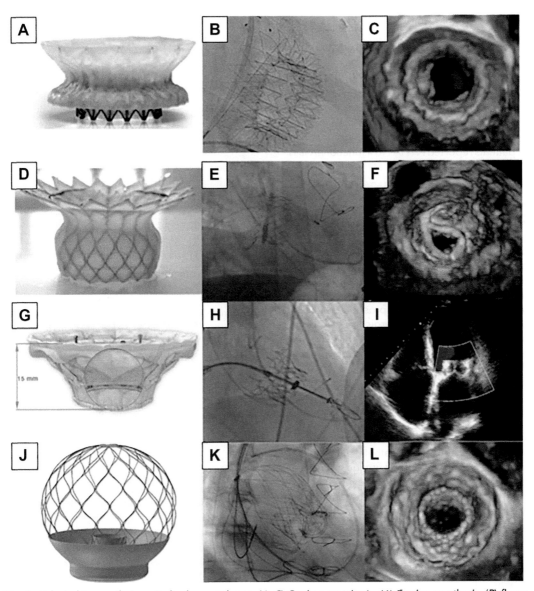

Fig. 4. Selected transcatheter mitral valve prostheses. (A–C) Cephea prosthesis. (A) Ex-vivo prosthesis, (B) fluoroscopic image of the valve, (C) 3-dimensional transesophageal echocardiography (3D-TEE) image from the left atrium. (D–F) Highlife valve. (D) Ex-vivo prosthesis, (E) fluoroscopic image of the valve, (F) 3D-TEE image from the left atrium. (G–I) Cardiovalve. (G) Ex-vivo prosthesis, (H) fluoroscopic image of the valve, (I) 3D-TEE image from the left atrium. (J–L) AltaValve. (J) Ex-vivo prosthesis, (K) fluoroscopic image of the valve, (L) 3D-TEE image from the left atrium. (Data from ([A-C] Alberto Alperi et al., Early Experience With a Novel Transfemoral Mitral Valve Implantation System in Complex Degenerative Mitral Regurgitation, JACC: Cardiovascular Interventions, 13 (20), 2020, 2427-2437, https://doi.org/10.1016/j.jcin.2020.08.006.); and ([D-F] Marco Barbanti et al., Transcatheter Mitral Valve Implantation Using the HighLife System, JACC: Cardiovascular Interventions, 10 (16), 2017, 1662-1670, https://doi.org/10.1016/j.jcin.2017.06.046.); and ([I] Francesco Maisano et al., 2-Year Follow-Up After Transseptal Transcatheter Mitral Valve Replacement With the Cardiovalve, JACC: Cardiovascular Interventions, 13 (17),2020, e163-e164, https://doi.org/10.1016/j.jcin.2020.05.032.); and ([J-L] Alfredo Nunes Ferreira-Neto et al. Transcatheter Mitral Valve Replacement With a New Supra-Annular Valve: First-in-Human Experience With the AltaValve System, JACC: Cardiovascular Interventions, 12 (2), 2019, 208-209, https://doi.org/10.1016/j.jcin.2018.10.056.))[34]

with a porcine pericardial valve.[20] It anchors using annular oversizing and a transapical tether. The D-shaped Tendyne prosthesis has a longer cuff specifically designed to orient toward the aortic-mitral curtain. Transapical access requires coaxial alignment with the center of the mitral annular orifice so that the tension from the apical cap maintains planar alignment with

the native annulus and the prosthesis does not
cant.

Two-year follow-up from an early cohort of 100
patients described a 1-year and 2-year mortality
rate of 27% (CI 19.2%–37%) and 41.6% (CI
32.2%–52.3%) respectively. Echocardiographic
follow-up found a 93.2% of none/trivial MR with
remainder of patients demonstrating mild MR.
Symptom improvement was significant as 81.6%
of patients reported NYHA I to II functional class.[32]

FUTURE DIRECTIONS

Prospective studies will determine the prosthesis
with best durability in terms of valve function
and PVL. Vulnerability to endocarditis is yet to
be determined. Late migration requiring revision
has been observed in some prostheses as well as
repairs for PVL.[29,32] Furthermore, understanding
the advantages transcatheter repair versus
replacement will need to be prospectively studied
and see if TEER emulates surgical repair for functional MR with late regurgitation.[33] Investigational
studies will hopefully answer questions regarding
the optimal thromboprophylaxis regiment and
duration.

SUMMARY

The complexities of mitral anatomy are testing the
limits of engineering transcatheter therapy. Itera-
tive advances in technology, imaging, and transcatheter technique have been key in developing
first-generation TMVR, and subsequent valves
will benefit from the lessons learned. Generaliz-
able therapy across broad populations has a high
bar to meet in terms of safety and efficacy given
the excellent performance of mitral TEER.

CLINICS CARE POINTS

- Transcatheter Mitral Valve Replacement
  (TMVR) is challenging due to the anatomic
  requirements of fitting a prosthesis, sealing
  and avoiding LVOT obstruction.

- Rigorous screening with 3D-CT is a necessary
  component for anatomic screening.

- Patients need to be suitable candidates for
  anticoagulation for TMVR and the optimal
  duration for anticoagualtion is not yet known.

DISCLOSURE

M.H. Eng is a clinical proctor for Edwards Lifesciences
and Medtronic. He is on the speaker's panel for
LivaNova. F. Zahr receives research and educational
grants and is a consultant for Edwards Lifesciences,
United States and Medtronic.

REFERENCES

1. Nkomo VT, Gardin JM, Skelton TN, et al. Burden of
   valvular heart diseases: a population-based study.
   Lancet 2006;368:1005–11.
2. Feldman T, Foster E, Glower DD, et al. Percutaneous repair or surgery for mitral regurgitation.
   N Engl J Med 2011;364:1395–406.
3. Stone GW, Lindenfeld J, Abraham WT, et al. Transcatheter Mitral-Valve Repair in Patients with Heart
   Failure. N Engl J Med 2018;379:2307–18.
4. Gavazzoni M, Taramasso M, Zuber M, et al.
   Conceiving MitraClip as a tool: percutaneous edge-
   to-edge repair in complex mitral valve anatomies.
   Eur Heart J Cardiovasc Imaging 2020;21:1059–67.
5. Thaden JJ, Malouf JF, Nkomo VT, et al. Mitral Valve
   Anatomic Predictors of Hemodynamic Success With
   Transcatheter Mitral Valve Repair. J Am Heart Assoc
   2018;7. https://doi.org/10.1161/jaha.117.007315.
6. Sorajja P, Kodali S, Reardon MJ, et al. Outcomes
   for the Commercial Use of Self-Expanding Prostheses in Transcatheter Aortic Valve Replacement: A
   Report From the STS/ACC TVT Registry. JACC Cardiovasc Interv 2017;10:2090–8.
7. Mack M, Carroll JD, Thourani V, et al. Transcatheter
   Mitral Valve Therapy in the United States: A Report
   From the STS-ACC TVT Registry. J Am Coll Cardiol
   2021;78:2326–53.
8. Van Mieghem NM, Piazza N, Anderson RH, et al.
   Anatomy of the Mitral Valvular Complex and Its Implications for Transcatheter Interventions for Mitral
   Regurgitation. J Am Coll Cardiol 2010;56:617–26.
9. Blanke P, Naoum C, Dvir D, et al. Predicting LVOT
   Obstruction in Transcatheter Mitral Valve Implantation: Concept of the Neo-LVOT. JACC Cardiovasc
   Imaging 2017;10:482–5.
10. Ben Ali W, Ludwig S, Duncan A, et al. Characteris-
    tics and outcomes of patients screened for trans-
    catheter mitral valve implantation: 1-year results
    from the CHOICE-MI registry. Eur J Heart Fail
    2022;24:887–98.
11. Tanawuttiwat T, O'Neill BP, Cohen MG, et al. New-
    onset atrial fibrillation after aortic valve replace-
    ment: comparison of transfemoral, transapical,
    transaortic, and surgical approaches. J Am Coll
    Cardiol 2014;63:1510–9.
12. Whisenant B, Kapadia SR, Eleid MF, et al. One-Year
    Outcomes of Mitral Valve-in-Valve Using the SA-
    PIEN 3 Transcatheter Heart Valve. JAMA Cardiol
    2020;5:1245–52.
13. Bapat V, Rajagopal V, Meduri C, et al. Early Experi-
    ence With New Transcatheter Mitral Valve Replace-
    ment. J Am Coll Cardiol 2018;71:12–21.

14. Wild MG, Kreidel F, Hell MM, et al. Transapical mitral valve implantation for treatment of symptomatic mitral valve disease: a real-world multicentre experience. Eur J Heart Fail 2022;24:899–907.

15. Kikoïne J, Himbert D, Chong-Nguyen C, et al. Incidence and Predictors of Early Major Bleeding After Transseptal Transcatheter Mitral Valve Replacement Using TAV. JACC Cardiovasc Interv 2023;16:2337–9.

16. Ludwig S, Perrin N, Coisne A, et al. Clinical outcomes of transcatheter mitral valve replacement: two-year results of the CHOICE-MI Registry. EuroIntervention 2023;19:512–25.

17. Fukui M, Sorajja P, Gossl M, et al. Left Ventricular Remodeling After Transcatheter Mitral Valve Replacement With Tendyne: New Insights From Computed Tomography. JACC Cardiovasc Interv 2020;13:2038–48.

18. Perl L, Kheifets M, Guido A, et al. Acute Reduction in Left Ventricular Function Following Transcatheter Mitral Edge to Edge Repair. J Am Heart Assoc 2023;12:e029735.

19. Eng MH, Kargoli F, Wang DD, et al. Short- and midterm outcomes in percutaneous mitral valve replacement using balloon expandable valves. Catheter Cardiovasc Interv 2021;98:1193–203.

20. Muller DWM, Farivar RS, Jansz P, et al. Transcatheter Mitral Valve Replacement for Patients With Symptomatic Mitral Regurgitation: A Global Feasibility Trial. J Am Coll Cardiol 2017;69:381–91.

21. Guerrero M, Wang DD, Eleid MF, et al. Prospective Study of TMVR Using Balloon-Expandable Aortic Transcatheter Valves in MAC: MITRAL Trial 1-Year Outcomes. JACC Cardiovasc Interv 2021;14:830–45.

22. Yoon SH, Bleiziffer S, Latib A, et al. Predictors of Left Ventricular Outflow Tract Obstruction After Transcatheter Mitral Valve Replacement. JACC Cardiovasc Interv 2019;12:182–93.

23. El Sabbagh A, Al-Hijji M, Wang DD, et al. Predictors of Left Ventricular Outflow Tract Obstruction After Transcatheter Mitral Valve Replacement in Severe Mitral Annular Calcification: An Analysis of the Transcatheter Mitral Valve Replacement in Mitral Annular Calcification Global Registry. Circ Cardiovasc Interv 2021;14:e010854.

24. Wang DD, Eng MH, Greenbaum A, et al. Predicting left ventricular outflow tract obstruction after transcatheter mitral valve replacement (TMVR): initial single center experience. JACC Cardiovasc Imaging 2016;11:1349–52.

25. Kohli K, Wei ZA, Sadri V, et al. Dynamic nature of the LVOT following transcatheter mitral valve replacement with LAMPOON: new insights from post-procedure imaging. Eur Heart J Cardiovasc Imaging 2022;23:650–62.

26. Meduri CU, Reardon MJ, Lim DS, et al. Novel Multiphase Assessment for Predicting Left Ventricular Outflow Tract Obstruction Before Transcatheter Mitral Valve Replacement. JACC Cardiovasc Interv 2019;12:2402–12.

27. Greenbaum AB, Condado JF, Eng M, et al. Long or redundant leaflet complicating transcatheter mitral valve replacement: Case vignettes that advocate for removal or reduction of the anterior mitral leaflet. Catheter Cardiovasc Interv 2018;92:627–32.

28. Yoon SH, Whisenant BK, Bleiziffer S, et al. Outcomes of transcatheter mitral valve replacement for degenerated bioprostheses, failed annuloplasty rings, and mitral annular calcification. Eur Heart J 2019;40:441–51.

29. Webb JG, Murdoch DJ, Boone RH, et al. Percutaneous Transcatheter Mitral Valve Replacement: First-in-Human Experience With a New Transseptal System. J Am Coll Cardiol 2019;73:1239–46.

30. Makkar RR, O'Neill W, Whisenant B, et al. Updated 30-Day Outcomes for the U.S. Early Feasibility Study of the SAPIEN M3 Transcatheter Mitral Valve Replacement System. J Am Coll Cardiol 2019;74:B8.

31. Zahr F, Song HK, Chadderdon S, et al. 1-Year Outcomes Following Transfemoral Transseptal Transcatheter Mitral Valve Replacement: Intrepid TMVR Early Feasibility Study Results. JACC Cardiovasc Interv 2023;16:2868–79.

32. Muller DWM, Sorajja P, Duncan A, et al. 2-Year Outcomes of Transcatheter Mitral Valve Replacement in Patients With Severe Symptomatic Mitral Regurgitation. J Am Coll Cardiol 2021;78:1847–59.

33. Acker MA, Parides MK, Perrault LP, et al. Mitral-valve repair versus replacement for severe ischemic mitral regurgitation. N Engl J Med 2014;370:23–32.

34. Alperi A, Granada JF, Bernier M, et al. Current Status and Future Prospects of Transcatheter Mitral Valve Replacement: JACC State-of-the-Art Review. J Am Coll Cardiol 2021;77:3058–78.

Transcatheter Mitral Valve Therapies in Patients with Mitral Annular Calcification

Patrick S. Kietrsunthorn, MD, Fadi Ghrair, MD,
Aaron R. Schelegle, MD, Jason R. Foerst, MD*

KEYWORDS

- Mitral annular calcification • Mitral valve stenosis • Mitral valve regurgitation
- Transcatheter mitral valve intervention

KEY POINTS

- MAC is a chronic progressive disease associated with significant morbidity and mortality.
- MAC poses considerable challenges for surgical and transcatheter mitral valve interventions.
- Novel dedicated TMVR devices are designed to overcome some of the challenges associated with transcatheter mitral valve interventions.
- Novel transcatheter electrosurgical techniques have been developed to overcome the disadvantages of transcatheter mitral valve interventions.

INTRODUCTION

Mitral annular calcification (MAC) is a chronic process involving degeneration and calcium deposition within the fibrous skeleton of the mitral valve annulus. It was first described in late 1908 by Bonniger[1] in its association with complete heart block. It can be asymptomatic, or it can have pathologic sequelae leading to cardiovascular morbidity and mortality. Its prevalence ranges from 8% to 42% based on multiple factors including the age and comorbidities of the studied population, and the diagnostic modality.[2–5]

Pathophysiology

The mitral valve annulus is a saddle-shaped structure. The anterior portion of the mitral valve annulus connects the anterior mitral valve leaflet (AMVL) to the aortic annulus, whereas the posterior mitral annulus connects the posterior mitral valve leaflet to the left atrial and left ventricular myocardium. The posterior mitral annulus is more dynamic than the anterior mitral annulus during the cardiac cycle, which might account

for the increased incidence of MAC developing in the posterior annulus.[6] Carpentier and colleagues[7] found that the calcification process remained localized to the annulus in 77%. The calcification involved more than one-third of the anulus in 88%, the full rim of the posterior anulus in 10.5%, and the whole anulus in 1.5%. The calcification process extended to the myocardial wall in 12% of the patients and to the papillary muscles in 4.5%.[7]

In the first decade of life, the mitral valve annulus consists of tightly packed thin collagen fibers. With age, the collagen fibers begin to degenerate with increased lipid and calcium deposits. In severe cases, large amorphous calcium globules are visible, separated by thick fibrous material.[8] More recently, calcified valvular pathologic specimens have shown features of bone formation (mature lamellar bone, endochondral bone, neoangiogenesis, osteoclast, and osteoblast activity) and inflammation (B and T lymphocytes). These findings suggest that MAC, in part, could be a result of chronic tissue degeneration and abnormal tissue repair.[9] In addition to

Structural and Interventional Cardiology, Virginia Tech Carilion School of Medicine and Carilion Clinic, 2001 Crystal Spring Road, Suite 203, Roanoke, VA 24014, USA
* Corresponding author.
E-mail address: jrfoerst@CarilionClinic.org

Intervent Cardiol Clin 13 (2024) 237–248
https://doi.org/10.1016/j.iccl.2024.01.002
2211-7458/24/© 2024 Elsevier Inc. All rights reserved.

histologic evidence of inflammation, there has been associations between MAC and blood inflammatory markers, such as C-reactive protein and interleukin-6.[10,11] Furthermore, new images from PET of the mitral valve annulus shows overlapping calcification and inflammation activity.[12]

Risk Factors

MAC shares similar risk factors with atherosclerotic disease, such as age, obesity, tobacco use, hypertension, and family history of myocardial infarction.[10] MAC is also associated with left ventricular hypertrophy and therefore is seen as a result of conditions that increase mitral valve stress (eg, hypertension, aortic valve stenosis, hypertrophic cardiomyopathy). Additionally, MAC is associated with chronic kidney disease. The association may be partly caused by abnormal calcium and phosphorus metabolism in this population.[13] Once diagnosed with MAC, diabetes and continued tobacco use are associated with greatest degree of MAC progression.[10]

MAC has also been associated with congenital connective tissue disorders, such as Marfan syndrome and Hurler syndrome.[14–16] Mitral valve prolapse is common in patients with Marfan syndrome and may be the cause of MAC because of increased stress. However, there may also be an association between the abnormal connective tissue composite to MAC development.[15] The association between Hurler syndrome and MAC may be explained by the abnormal fibroblasts and collagen degeneration that is seen in these patients.[16]

Lastly, female sex has been associated with MAC. Even though the prevalence of MAC may be similar between males and females of the same age, the degree of calcium deposition seems to be more severe in females.[4,10,17,18] This association may be partly attributed to calcium deposits secondary to severe bone loss in postmenopausal females with osteoporosis.[19]

Diagnosis and Classification

MAC is often first detected by two-dimensional transthoracic echocardiography (TTE). This modality also allows for assessment of mitral valvular function to determine the severity of mitral valve stenosis (MS) and/or mitral valve regurgitation (MR) when present. There is no consensus regarding the grading of MAC severity by echocardiography. In the past, studies have graded MAC in terms of the extent of circumferential calcification (mild < one-third involved, moderate < half involved, severe > half involved).[20,21] However, this grading system has not been linked to any clinical outcomes. Accurate classification of MAC severity by TTE is difficult because of the lack of spatial resolution that is required.

Cardiac computed tomography (CT) has become the gold standard for quantitative and qualitative assessment of MAC. Guerrero and colleagues[22] devised a CT-based MAC classification system to predict bioprosthetic valvular migration/embolization after transcatheter mitral valve replacement (TMVR) with an Edwards SAPIEN valve (Fig. 1).

Caseous calcification of the mitral annulus (CCMA) is considered a rare variant of MAC (Fig. 2A–E). The prevalence of CCMA is less than 0.1% in the general population and approximately 2.7% of patients with MAC. CCMA usually appears as a round echodense mitral annular mass with an echolucent center. This unusual appearance shares similarities to cardiac tumors and abscess and can easily lead to misdiagnosis. CCMA poses additional challenges for management compared with traditional MAC. This "toothpaste" MAC usually involves a large portion of the atrioventricular (AV) groove and ventricular myocardium, which has a higher risk of AV groove disruption and perforation from aggressive debridement. Partial debridement and unroofing procedure are not advisable because it promotes continuous exposure of the systemic circulation with necrotic debris. Lastly, CCMA is a dynamic process and can recur even after successful surgical excision.[23]

Clinical Impact and Prognosis

The Northern Manhattan Study found that MAC was an independent predictor of cardiovascular

Points	Calcium thickness (mm)	Calcium distribution	Trigone involvement	Leaflet involvement	MAC score	Valve migration/embolization (%)
0	-	-	None	None	≤6	60
1	≤5	<180 degree	1	1	7	12.5
2	5–9.9	180-270 degrees	2	2	8	8.7
3	≥10	>270 degrees	-	-	≥9	0

Fig. 1. MAC scoring system derived by Guerrero and colleagues.

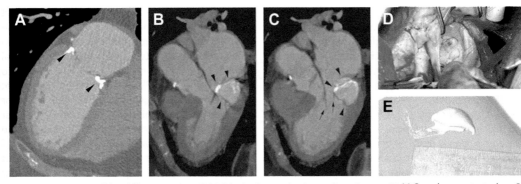

Fig. 2. Comparison of the different types of MAC including caseating or "toothpaste" MAC as demonstrated on CT. (A) Traditional MAC on cardiac CT (*arrowheads*). (B, C) Mitral valve leaflets (*arrow*) and caseous calcification of the mitral annulus on cardiac CT (*arrowheads*). (D) Intraoperative photograph demonstrating the caseous calcification after incision. (E) Pasty white material was subsequently aspirated. (Elgendy, I.Y. and Conti, C.R. (2013), Caseous Calcification of the Mitral Annulus: A Review. Clin Cardiol, 36: E27-E31. https://doi.org/10.1002/clc.22199.)

events, specifically myocardial infarction and vascular death. The association is proportional to the severity of MAC with the strongest association to MAC greater than 4-mm thick measured on M-mode echocardiography.[24]

In addition to cardiovascular disease and cardiovascular death, the Framingham cohort also found a correlation between MAC and all-cause mortality with approximately a 10% increase in all-cause mortality for each 1 mm of MAC.[25]

The Framingham cohort showed a relationship between MAC and stroke even after adjusting for classical risk of ischemic vascular events (including calcification, age, sex, hypertension, diabetes mellitus, tobacco use, coronary heart disease, and congestive heart failure). Additionally, there was a continuous relationship between the severity of MAC (defined by the thickness on M-mode echocardiography) and the relative risk of stroke.[26] The risk of stroke in relation to MAC may be partly explained by the increased risk of left atrial enlargement and subsequent atrial fibrillation in this population.[27] Additionally, there are cases demonstrating residual thrombotic material on calcified nodules of the mitral annulus in patients with ischemic strokes with no other definitive cause.[28]

Lastly, in small studies, MAC has been implemented as a potential nidus for bacterial endocarditis and nonbacterial thromboembolic events. Specifically, *Staphylococcus aureus* has been associated with lesions located on the calcified mitral annulus, whereas streptococcal infections are associated with lesions located on the leaflets.[29]

Mechanism of Mitral Valve Dysfunction

MAC is an uncommon cause of mitral valvular disfunction. Nonetheless, MAC has been associated with MR and MS.[30] A large retrospective study of 24,380 echocardiograms found that MAC was present in 11.7% of patients with MR and only in 4.3% of patients without MR.[31] The mitral annulus is a dynamic structure that contracts and relaxes with the cardiac cycle; the decrease in dynamic annular motion with MAC may partly account for the development of MR.[32]

MAC is a rare cause of MS because the calcification is often confined to the annulus and does not involve the commissures or the leaflets. However, in severe cases, calcifications of the commissures and the leaflet may be present. Specifically, MS has been associated with calcification and reduced mobility of the AMVL.[33]

SURGICAL MANAGEMENT OF MITRAL ANNULAR CALCIFICATION WITH VALVULAR DYSFUNCTION

Uncomplicated MAC that does not affect mitral valve function is managed conservatively with risk factor modification and periodic follow-up imaging. However, complicated MAC causing valvular dysfunction (regurgitation, stenosis, or mixed pathology) may require further invasive interventions. The main strategies for managing mitral valve dysfunction accompanying MAC are surgical interventions and transcatheter interventions. Comprehensive evaluation by a dedicated multidisciplinary heart team with special expertise in MAC is recommended.

Classic surgical repair or replacement usually starts with an en-block excision of the annular calcium followed by reconstruction of the annulus to be use as the anchor point for repair/replacement. Mitral annular reconstruction carries the risk of injury to the left circumflex (LCx) artery, AV groove disruption, and calcium embolization.[7,34] The risk of these complications increases with the extent of calcification, especially if the ventricular myocardium is involved. Ultrasonic debridement is a calcium modification technique that is used for dense calcification. It allows adequate MAC modification to properly seat and suture a bioprosthesis while minimizing annular manipulation, which in turn reduces the risk of LCx artery injury, AV groove disruption, and calcium embolization.[35] A surgical repair strategy is usually feasible in cases of mitral valve prolapse with MAC. In this situation, the anterior mitral valve can be repaired with chordal transfer/shortening and the posterior leaflet can be repaired with triangular/quadrangular resection with or without chordal shortening. Once the appropriate valvular repair is completed, the valve is sutured to the reconstructed annulus and reinforced by a prosthetic ring on the atrial side. In cases not feasible for repair, replacement is performed by suturing the prosthetic valve to the decalcified and reconstructed annulus.[7,34]

To minimize complications associated with decalcification of MAC, several alternative techniques have been described. One option is to leave the annular calcium intact and place sutures deep to the calcium. This technique increases the risk of LCx injury and may not allow for proper bioprosthesis seating (resulting in paravalvular leak [PVL]) but can potentially reduce the risk of AV groove disruption.[36] Another option is to place an intra-atrial prosthesis by adding a Dacron collar to the prosthesis and suturing the collar to the atrial wall. This approach is effective for MR but not for MS because the atrial bioprosthesis does not alleviate the native mitral valve obstruction. This particular technique may increase the risk of atrial dissection and bleeding in the portion of the atrial myocardium that is exposed to left ventricular pressure.[37] Lastly, mitral valve bypass may be performed for MS (but not effective for MR). In this case, a conduit is placed from the left atrial appendage or left atrial atriotomy site to the left ventricular apex. A bioprosthetic or mechanical valve is placed in the conduit close to the ventricular apex attachment to reduce exposure of the conduit to left ventricular pressure. This approach reduces time of cardiopulmonary bypass and manipulation of MAC at the cost of potential conduit failure and/or thrombosis.[38]

Surgical implantation of transcatheter valve in native mitral annular calcification has been described using a transatrial surgical mitral valve replacement with a SAPIEN 3 transcatheter valve. This approach offers several advantages over conventional surgical and transcatheter approaches. This technique requires minimal MAC manipulation, which reduces the risk associated with traditional surgical debridement. The direct visualization of the mitral valve allows for precise balloon sizing and bioprosthetic valve anchoring with pledgeted sutures (of the native mitral leaflet to the skirt of the SAPIEN 3 valve) to reduce the risk of PVL and valve embolization. To further reduce the risk of PVL, the operator can perform commissural plication to better approximate the D-shape native annulus to the circular SAPIEN valve. Lastly, this approach allows for resection of the AMVL (with or without septal myectomy) to prevent left ventricular outflow tract (LVOT) obstruction.[39–41]

TRANSCATHETER MANAGEMENT OF MITRAL ANNULAR CALCIFICATION WITH VALVULAR DYSFUNCTION

Transcatheter valve implantation offers an alternative option for patients who are at high or prohibitive surgical risk. Transcatheter techniques specifically avoid risks associated with aorta cross-clamp, cardiopulmonary bypass, AV groove disruption, and LCx injury. Mortality of surgical management of MAC is reported to be 3.3% to 5.8% with a 5-year mortality rate of 60%.[7,34] Initially, transcatheter valvular implantation was performed using a transapical approach. With the advancement of transseptal techniques, transseptal approach has gained popularity because of its potential reduction in bleeding risk, lower 30-day mortality, lower 1-year mortality, and shorter in-hospital stay.[42,43]

Off-Label Use of SAPIEN in Mitral Annular Calcification

Most transseptal TMVR in MAC has been performed using the SAPIEN XT or SAPIEN 3 valve, which was originally designed for a circular aortic annulus. The MITRAL trial is the first prospective trial evaluating the use of balloon-expandable aortic transcatheter heart valves (THVs) through the transseptal approach in the mitral position for valve-in-MAC, valve-in-ring, and valve-in-valve. The trial showed improvement in symptoms, improvement in quality of life, and stable prosthesis function at 2-year follow-up.[44] The major concerns of using the circular SAPIEN valves in the D-shaped mitral annulus are PVL and prosthesis migration/embolization, which has fueled the need for dedicated TMVR devices.[45]

Dedicated Transcatheter Mitral Valve Replacement Devices Under Investigation for Mitral Annular Calcification

The Tendyne valve system (Abbott Structural) has been evaluated for treatment of patients with MR and is currently being evaluated in patients with MAC (Fig. 3A). The valve consists of an inner porcine trileaflet valve that is inside an outer D-shaped nitinol self-expanding stent (designed to match the shape of the mitral annulus). The prosthesis is attached to an ultrahigh-molecular-weight tether and an apical pad that anchors the valve to the apex of the left ventricle. The system is delivered via a left anterolateral thoracotomy and a 36F catheter transapical sheath. Early outcome of the Tendyne valve in MAC shows improved symptoms as measured by the New York Heart Association functional class and the Kansas City Cardiomyopathy Questionnaire.[46,47] The SUMMIT trial is an ongoing randomized clinical trial comparing the Tendyne valve with transcatheter edge-edge repair (MitraClip) with a separate non-randomized arm for patients with severe MAC.[48]

The SAPIEN M3 TMVR system (Edwards Lifesciences) is a balloon expandable 29-mm bioprosthetic valve in a nitinol docking system (Fig. 3C–E). The SAPIEN M3 is modified from the SAPIEN 3 valve to have a full frame skirt to reduce regurgitant flow around the frame and docking system. The docking system encircles the native mitral valve leaflet to provide a landing zone for the valve. The system is delivered through a 28F catheter steerable sheath via the transseptal approach. The early feasibility completed in 2018 and updated in 2019 showed

reduction in MR severity and improvement in symptoms.[49] The ENCIRCLE trial is an ongoing nonrandomized trial to evaluate clinical outcome of the SAPIEN M3 TMVR system for MR with a separate arm for patients with MAC (Fig. 7).[50]

The Intrepid TMVR system (Medtronic) is a 27-mm bioprosthetic valve that is seated inside a 42-mm or 48-mm outer stent, which is designed to engage and conform to the mitral valve leaflet and annulus while preserving the circular shape of the inner valve (see Fig. 3B). The valve is delivered via a 35F catheter system using a transseptal approach. It completed its early feasibility trial for MR in 2022.[51] The APOLLO trial is an ongoing nonrandomized trial to evaluate clinical outcome of the Intrepid valve for MR with a separate arm for patients with MAC.[52]

CHALLENGES ASSOCIATED WITH TRANSCATHETER MITRAL VALVE REPLACEMENT

Paravalvular Leak

PVL is a common complication of TMVR, especially in the era of balloon expandable valve-in-MAC. The circular SAPIEN valve does not completely approximate the D-shaped mitral annulus. This can result in commissural leaks, especially if the native valve has baseline commissural regurgitation jets. Additionally, the degree of MAC (even though important in anchoring of the THV) can result in PVL because the calcified annulus is less

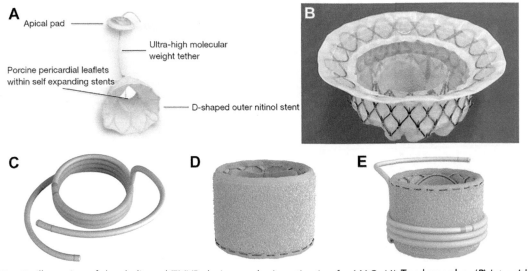

Fig. 3. Illustration of the dedicated TMVR devices under investigation for MAC. (*A*) Tendyne valve. (*B*) Intrepid valve. (*C–E*) SAPIEN M3 system. ([A] Beller JP, Rogers JH, Thourani VH. Ailawadi G. Early clinical results with the Tendyne transcatheter mitral valve replacement system. Ann Cardiothorac Surg 2018:7(6):776-779. https://doi.org/10.21037/acs.2018.10.01; [B] Images used with permission from Medtronic, plc © 2024; [C-E] John G. Webb et al., Percutaneous Transcatheter Mitral Valve Replacement: First-in-Human Experience With a New Transseptal System, Journal of the American College of Cardiology, 73 (11), 2019, 1239-1246, https://doi.org/10.1016/j.jacc.2018.12.065.)

likely to conform to the circular shape of the THV.[53] PVL are usually clinically silent; however, in severe cases, patients may present with signs and symptoms of decompensated heart failure and hemolytic anemia.[54] Severe PVL is treated with a transcatheter closure with off-label occluder devices (illustrative case in Fig. 4A–F). The challenge of this procedure is the crossing and delivery of equipment across the defect. Once deployed, the device can also interfere with valve function and cause worsening regurgitation or stenosis.[55]

Transcatheter Heart Valve Migration and Embolization

The risk of valve migration/embolization is high in TMVR because of the D-shaped annulus and the dynamic motion of the annulus throughout the cardiac cycle. Studies report incidence of migration/embolization rates ranging from 8.6% up to 60% (in patients with high-risk features). The MAC score is used to help predict the risk of valve migration/embolization to guide management strategies (see Fig. 1).[22] Valve migration can occur acutely postdeployment or subacutely over time leading to atrialization of the THV and transvalvular regurgitation (illustrative case in Fig. 5A–F). Newer dedicated transcatheter mitral valves are designed with a more robust tethering mechanism to mitigate this risk, such as the Tendyne valve and the SAPIEN M3 system (as detailed previously).

Left Ventricular Outflow Tract Obstruction

The risk of LVOT obstruction is another major disadvantage of transcatheter valve implantation. Unlike surgical mitral valve replacement, TMVR does not allow for resection of the native AMVL resulting in an increased risk of LVOT obstruction.[56] In one study, the risk of LVOT obstruction with hemodynamic compromise occurred in 11.2% of patients receiving the balloon expandable SAPIEN 3 in MAC. If LVOT obstruction occurs, it carries an extremely high mortality rate of up to 70% at 30 days and 85% at 1 year (Fig. 6).[57] Two potential mechanisms of LVOT obstruction have been described: fixed obstruction from the AMVL being shifted toward the interventricular septum, and dynamic obstruction from systolic anterior motion of the shifted AMVL.[58] A fixed LVOT obstruction is predicted by using multislice cardiac CT to create the "neo-LVOT" (the predicted LVOT area post-TMVR between the ventricular septum and the shifted AMVL) or the "skirt neo-LVOT" (the predicted LVOT area post-TMVR between the

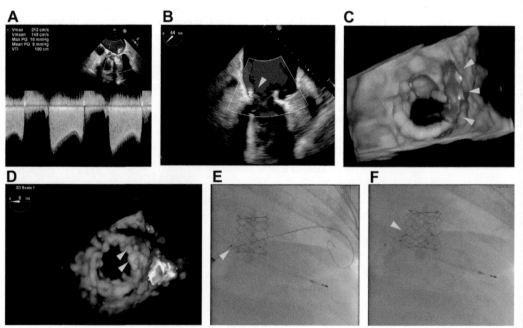

Fig. 4. A 74-year-old woman with severe mitral stenosis in the setting of MAC who presents for valve-in-MAC (29-mm SAPIEN 3) with resulting PVL successfully treated with two AVP II plug (8 mm and 12 mm). (A) Pre-TMVR Doppler of the mitral valve showing severe mitral valve stenosis. (B) Post-TMVR color Doppler showing paravalvular leak (*arrowhead*) of the 29-mm SAPIEN 3 valve. (C) Three-dimensional image post-TMVR with the SAPIEN 3 valve with significant PVL (*arrowheads*). (D) Three-dimensional image of the SAPIEN 3 valve with two AVP II plugs (*arrowheads*) and no residual PVL. (E) Deployment of the first AVP II plug (*arrowhead*). (F) Deployment of the second AVP II plug (*arrowhead*).

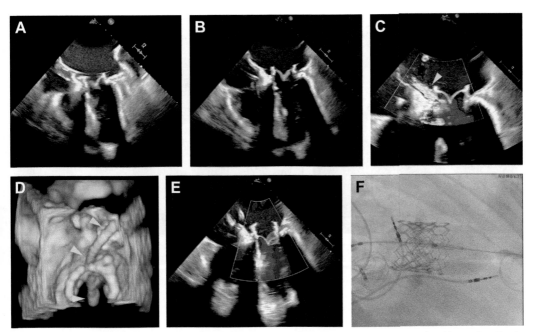

Fig. 5. A 76-year-old woman with severe mitral stenosis in the setting of MAC s/p TMVR with a 29-mm SAPIEN 3 at 15 months prior who presents with valve migration toward the left atrium resulting in transvalvular regurgitation through the atrialized uncovered valve frame successfully treated with valve-in-valve TMVR. (*A*) Final midesophageal transesophageal echocardiography image after her initial TMVR 15 months ago. (*B*) Current midesophageal transesophageal echocardiography image showing atrial migration of the THV compared with prior image. (*C*) Color Doppler showing severe transvalvular regurgitation (*arrowhead*). (*D*) Three-dimensional transesophageal echocardiography surgeon view of the mitral valve with the glide wire (*arrowheads*) crossing through the stent frame. (*E*) After valve-in-valve TMVR with trace residual transvalvular regurgitation. (*F*) Fluoroscopic image of the valve-in-valve deployment.

ventricular septum and the THV skirt). A neo-LVOT area of less than 170 to 190 mm^2 can predict an increased risk of post-TMVR LVOT obstruction.[59] Keep in mind that the actual neo-LVOT may be different from the predicted neo-LVOT depending on the final depth of valve implant (which may be difficult to control depending on patient anatomy). Dynamic LVOT obstruction is more difficult to predict and depends on various parameters including aorto-mitral angulation, mitral annulus-interventricular septum distance, ventricular septal wall thickness, anterior mitral leaflet length, and mitral chordae redundancy.[58]

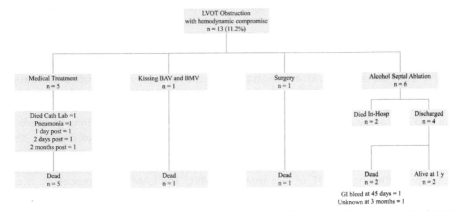

Fig. 6. Mortality breakdown of LVOT obstruction post-TMVR from Mitral Trial. GI, gastrointestinal. BAV, balloon aortic valvuloplasty. BMV, balloon mitral valvuloplasty. (Mayra Guerrero et al. 1-Year Outcomes of Transcatheter Mitral Valve Replacement in Patients With Severe Mitral Annular Calcification, Journal of the American College of Cardiology, 71 (17), 2018, 1841-1853, https://doi.org/10.1016/j.jacc.2018.02.054.)

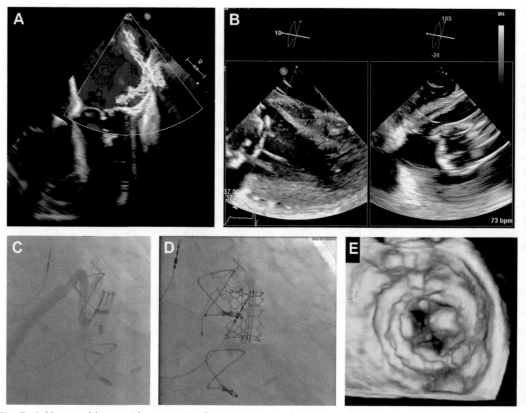

Fig. 7. A 80-year-old men with severe mitral regurgitation in the setting of dense circumferential mitral annular calcification treated with a 29 mm Edwards SAPIEN M3 valve and the SAPIEN M3 dock. (*A*) Pre-procedure transesophageal echocardiogram showing severe eccentric mitral valve regurgitation. (*B*) Transgastric view of the transesophageal echocardiogram showing the SAPIEN M3 dock positioned around the mitral valve apparatus. (*C*) Fluoroscopic imaging of the SAPIEN M3 dock being delivered. Note the severe circumferential mitral annular calcification. (*D*) Fluoroscopic imaging of the 29 mm Edwards SAPIEN M3 value deployed in the SAPIEN M3 dock. (*E*) 3D transesophageal imaging of the 29 mm Edwards SAPIEN M3 value deployed in the SAPIEN M3 dock.

Alcohol septal ablation

Alcohol septal ablation (ASA) is performed to reduce the risk of LVOT obstruction. ASA is performed by isolating a septal perforator branch with an over-the-wire coronary balloon, confirming isolation of the desired septal myocardium under TTE guidance with injection of an echocardiographic contrast agent, and administration of 1 to 3 mL of 98% dehydrated alcohol at a rate of 1 mL/min. ASA works by reducing septal wall thickness and increasing the distance between the ventricular septum to the shifted AMVL. ASA is done preemptively or as a bail-out procedure. When done preemptively for patients with a predicted neo-LVOT of less than 189 mm^2, there was an average increased LVOT area of 111.2 mm^2 from the predicted neo-LVOT. Patients who underwent ASA are at elevated risk of high-grade AV block requiring pacemaker implantation.[60,61]

Laceration of the Anterior Mitral Leaflet to Prevent Outflow Obstruction

The laceration of the anterior mitral leaflet to prevent outflow obstruction (LAMPOON) procedure is designed as an alternative to surgical resection of the AMVL. To reduce the risk of LVOT obstruction, the AMVL is split down the middle with radiofrequency energy to alleviate any obstruction. The procedure requires two access sites, one for the radiofrequency wire and the other for the snare. Once the wire is passed through the base of the AMVL at the appropriate position, the wire is snared and both systems are carefully withdrawn while applying radiofrequency energy to split the AMVL. The LAMPOON procedure is performed from an anterograde approach or a retrograde approach. The anterograde approach involves two transseptal punctures from the femoral vein, whereas the retrograde is done through femoral artery access. The retrograde approach is more straightforward because the orientation of the aorta/LVOT is aligned with the AMVL. However, the retrograde approach is contraindicated in the presence of a mechanical aortic valve prosthesis. The anterograde approach is performed in patients with a mechanical aortic valve prosthesis, but the AMVL is not usually aligned with the transseptal site and careful catheter positioning is required to avoid eccentric splitting of the AMVL. In cases where the base of the mitral valve is protected (eg, post-TMVR), a rescue modified LAMPOON procedure is performed by splitting the AMVL from the tip to the base using the frame of the THV as a backstop (Fig. 8).[58] Appropriate preprocedure assessment of the neo-LVOT and the "skirt neo-LVOT" is necessary to determine if the patient will benefit. Because the LAMPOON procedure does not address the skirt of the THV, the resulting LVOT after splitting the AMVL is bordered by the skirt of the THV and the interventricular septum (skirt neo-LVOT). The LAMPOON procedure only benefits patients with a low neo-LVOT area but an adequate skirt neo-LVOT area. In cases where the skirt neo-LVOT area is also low, the LAMPOON procedure is not effective at addressing the LVOT obstruction.

Septal Scoring Along the Midline Endocardium

The septal scoring along the midline endocardium (SESAME) procedure is designed as an alternative for surgical septal myectomy. It was initially intended for treatment of patients with hypertrophic cardiomyopathy but has been adapted for treatment of TMVR-associated LVOT obstruction. To reduce the septal thickness at the LVOT, a guidewire is used to mechanically enter the basal portion of the LVOT septum and exits past the

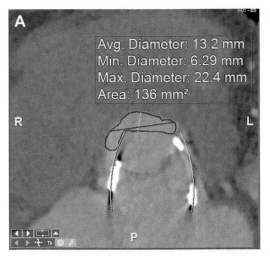
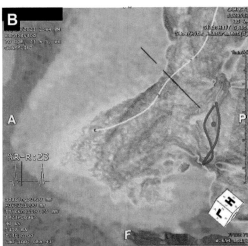
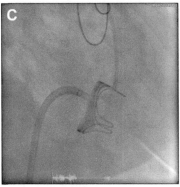
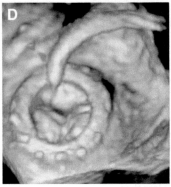
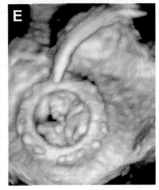

Fig. 8. A 73-year-old woman with history of surgical mitral valve replacement (29 mm Edwards Thermafix pericardial bioprosthesis) who presents with severe bioprosthetic mitral valve stenosis (mean gradient 13 mmHg and calculated valve area of 0.7 cm². (A, B) Computed tomography neo-LVOT reconstruction with an embedded 29 mm Edwards SAPIEN 3 Ultra RESILIA valve showing a calculated neo-LVOT of 136 mm². (C) Fluoroscopic positioning of the LAMPOON system with the "flying-V" at the tip of anterior bioprosthetic mitral valve leaflet. (D) Transesophageal echocardiogram positioning of the LAMPOON system at the tip of the anterior bioprosthetic mitral valve leaflet. (E) Transesophageal echocardiogram after tip-to-base LAMPOON demonstrating successful laceration of the anterior bioprosthetic mitral valve leaflet at the midline with resulting flail anterior bioprosthetic mitral valve leaflet.

hypertrophied myocardium. Once proper wire trajectory and placement is confirmed, the tip is snared, and the myocardium is splayed open using radiofrequency energy.[62] The first-in-human report was published in May of 2022 with a post-procedure LVOT area 102 mm^2 higher than the predicted neo-LVOT.[63] The SESAME procedure is particularly beneficial in patients who lack a suitable septal perforator artery for ASA and a low predicted skirt neo-LVOT area.

SUMMARY

MAC is a pathologic entity that is getting increasingly recognized with the advancement of diagnostic imaging modalities, especially in an era with a growing elderly population. When present, it can affect the decision-making process in managing concomitant mitral valvular disease. Multiple surgical and transcatheter techniques have been developed to overcome these challenges. Further advancement in transcatheter technology offers promising minimally invasive solutions for this patient population who often has prohibitive surgical risk.

CLINICS CARE POINTS

- MAC poses considerable challenges for both surgical and transcatheter mitral valve intervention. As such, it is important to identify the presence of MAC when evaluating patients with mitral valve dysfunction.

- Due to the challenges of mitral valve intervention, patient who have symptomatic mitral valve dysfunction associated with MAC should undergo aggressive medical management as the first line treatment. Initial medical management should be directed towards other co-morbidities that could affect the severity of mitral valvular dysfunction such as heart failure, hypertension, LVOT obstruction, Aortic stenosis, etc.

- For patients who have refractory symptomatic mitral valve dysfunction associated with MAC being considered for transcatheter mitral valve intervention, the neo-LVOT should be predicted. LVOT modification should be considered if the neo-LVOT is less than 190 mm^2 and is strongly recommended if less than 150 mm^2.

- Patients with symptomatic mitral valve dysfunction and MAC should be referred to a tertiary care center with a dedicated heart team with expertise to manage complex mitral valve disease.

DISCLOSURES

Dr J.R. Foerst is a consultant for Medtronic and Edwards Lifesciences.

REFERENCES

1. Bonniger, M. Bluttransfusion bei pernizioser anamie: (b) Zwei Falle von Herzblock.
2. Allison MA, Cheung P, Criqui MH, et al. Mitral and aortic annular calcification are highly associated with systemic calcified atherosclerosis. Circulation 2006;113(6):861–6.
3. Barasch E, Gottdiener JS, Marino Larsen EK, et al. Clinical significance of calcification of the fibrous skeleton of the heart and aortosclerosis in community dwelling elderly. The Cardiovascular Health Study (CHS). Am Heart J 2006;151(1):39–47.
4. Kanjanauthai S, Nasir K, Katz R, et al. Relationships of mitral annular calcification to cardiovascular risk factors: the Multi-Ethnic Study of Atherosclerosis (MESA). Atherosclerosis 2010;213(2):558–62.
5. Massera D, Kizer JR, Dweck MR. Mechanisms of mitral annular calcification. Trends Cardiovasc Med 2020;30(5):289–95.
6. Dal-Bianco JP, Levine RA. Anatomy of the mitral valve apparatus: role of 2D and 3D echocardiography. Cardiol Clin 2013;31(2):151–64.
7. Carpentier AF, Pellerin M, Fuzellier JF, et al. Extensive calcification of the mitral valve anulus: pathology and surgical management. J Thorac Cardiovasc Surg 1996;111(4):718–30.
8. Sell S, Scully RE. Aging changes in the aortic and mitral valves. Histologic and histochemical studies, with observations on the pathogenesis of calcific aortic stenosis and calcification of the mitral annulus. Am J Pathol 1965;46(3):345–65.
9. Mohler ER, Gannon F, Reynolds C, et al. Bone formation and inflammation in cardiac valves. Circulation 2001;103(11):1522–8.
10. Elmariah S, Budoff MJ, Delaney JAC, et al. Risk factors associated with the incidence and progression of mitral annulus calcification: the Multi-Ethnic Study of Atherosclerosis. Am Heart J 2013;166(5):904–12.
11. Thanassoulis G, Massaro JM, Cury R, et al. Associations of long-term and early adult atherosclerosis risk factors with aortic and mitral valve calcium. J Am Coll Cardiol 2010;55(22):2491–8.
12. Massera D, Trivieri MG, Andrews JPM, et al. Disease activity in mitral annular calcification. Circ Cardiovasc Imaging 2019;12(2):e008513.
13. Elmariah S, Delaney JAC, Bluemke DA, et al. Associations of LV hypertrophy with prevalent and incident valve calcification: Multi-Ethnic Study of Atherosclerosis. JACC Cardiovasc Imaging 2012;5(8):781–8.

14. Horiuchi K. Mitral annular calcification in Marfan syndrome: a 38-year follow-up observation. Thorac Cardiovasc Surg Rep 2021;10(1):e49–51.

15. Radke RM, Baumgartner H. Diagnosis and treatment of Marfan syndrome: an update. Heart Br Card Soc 2014;100(17):1382–91.

16. Schieken RM, Kerber RE, Ionasescu VV, et al. Cardiac manifestations of the mucopolysaccharidoses. Circulation 1975;52(4):700–5.

17. Boon A, Cheriex E, Lodder J, et al. Cardiac valve calcification: characteristics of patients with calcification of the mitral annulus or aortic valve. Heart Br Card Soc 1997;78(5):472–4.

18. Roberts WC. Morphologic features of the normal and abnormal mitral valve. Am J Cardiol 1983; 51(6):1005–28.

19. Sugihara N, Matsuzaki M. The influence of severe bone loss on mitral annular calcification in postmenopausal osteoporosis of elderly Japanese women. Jpn Circ J 1993;57(1):14–26.

20. Van Hemelrijck M, Taramasso M, Gülmez G, et al. Mitral annular calcification: challenges and future perspectives. Indian J Thorac Cardiovasc Surg Off Organ Assoc Thorac Cardiovasc Surg India 2020; 36(4):397–403.

21. Abudiab MM, Chebrolu LH, Schutt RC, et al. Doppler echocardiography for the estimation of LV filling pressure in patients with mitral annular calcification. JACC Cardiovasc Imaging 2017; 10(12):1411–20.

22. Guerrero M, Wang DD, Pursnani A, et al. A cardiac computed tomography-based score to categorize mitral annular calcification severity and predict valve embolization. JACC Cardiovasc Imaging 2020;13(9):1945–57.

23. Elgendy IY, Conti CR. Caseous calcification of the mitral annulus: a review. Clin Cardiol 2013;36(10): E27–31.

24. Kohsaka S, Jin Z, Rundek T, et al. Impact of mitral annular calcification on cardiovascular events in a multiethnic community. The Northern Manhattan Study. JACC Cardiovasc Imaging 2008;1(5):617–23.

25. Fox CS, Vasan RS, Parise H, et al. Mitral annular calcification predicts cardiovascular morbidity and mortality: the Framingham Heart Study. Circulation 2003;107(11):1492–6.

26. Mitral Annular Calcification and the Risk of Stroke in an Elderly Cohort | NEJM https://www.nejm.org/doi/full/10.1056/nejm199208063270602. Accessed July 5, 2023.

27. Fox CS, Parise H, Vasan RS, et al. Mitral annular calcification is a predictor for incident atrial fibrillation. Atherosclerosis 2004;173(2):291–4.

28. Eicher JC, Soto FX, DeNadai L, et al. Possible association of thrombotic, nonbacterial vegetations of the mitral ring-mitral annular calcium and stroke. Am J Cardiol 1997;79(12):1712–5.

29. Pressman GS, Rodriguez-Ziccardi M, Gartman CH, et al. Mitral annular calcification as a possible nidus for endocarditis: a descriptive series with bacteriological differences noted. J Am Soc Echocardiogr Off Publ Am Soc Echocardiogr 2017;30(6):572–8.

30. Labovitz AJ, Nelson JG, Windhorst DM, et al. Frequency of mitral valve dysfunction from mitral annular calcium as detected by Doppler echocardiography. Am J Cardiol 1985;55(1):133–7.

31. Movahed MR, Saito Y, Ahmadi-Kashani M, et al. Mitral annulus calcification is associated with valvular and cardiac structural abnormalities. Cardiovasc Ultrasound 2007;5:14.

32. Pressman GS, Movva R, Topilsky Y, et al. Mitral annular dynamics in mitral annular calcification: a three-dimensional imaging study. J Am Soc Echocardiogr Off Publ Am Soc Echocardiogr 2015; 28(7):786–94.

33. Muddassir SM, Pressman GS. Mitral annular calcification as a cause of mitral valve gradients. Int J Cardiol 2007;123(1):58–62.

34. El-Eshmawi A, Alexis SL, Sengupta A, et al. Surgical management of mitral annular calcification. Curr Opin Cardiol 2020;35(2):107–15.

35. Brescia AA, Rosenbloom LM, Watt TMF, et al. Ultrasonic emulsification of severe mitral annular calcification during mitral valve replacement. Ann Thorac Surg 2022;113(6):2092–6.

36. Cammack PL, Edie RN, Henry Edmunds L. Bar calcification of the mitral anulus: a risk factor in mitral valve operations. J Thorac Cardiovasc Surg 1987; 94(3):399–404.

37. Mihos CG, Santana O, Peguero J, et al. Intra-atrial placement of a mitral prosthesis in patients with severe mitral annular calcification. J Heart Valve Dis 2012;21(6):702–6.

38. Said SM, Schaff HV. An alternate approach to valve replacement in patients with mitral stenosis and severely calcified annulus. J Thorac Cardiovasc Surg 2014;147(6):e76–8.

39. Albacker TB, Bakir B, Eldemerdash A, et al. Surgical mitral valve replacement using direct implantation of Sapien 3 valve in a patients with severe mitral annular calcification without adjunctive techniques, a case report. J Cardiothorac Surg 2020;15(1):42.

40. Hamid UI, Gregg A, Ball P, et al. Open transcatheter valve implantation for mitral annular calcification: one-year outcomes. JTCVS Tech 2021;10:254–61.

41. Kobsa S, Sorabella RA, Eudailey K, et al. Transatrial implantation of the Sapien 3 heart valve in severe mitral annular calcification: multi-clinic experience, written and video description. Struct Heart 2019; 3(1):74–6.

42. Nazir S, Lohani S, Tachamo N, et al. Outcomes following transcatheter transseptal versus transapical mitral valve-in-valve and valve-in-ring procedures. J Cardiovasc Thorac Res 2018;10(4):182–6.

43. Al-Tawil M, Butt S, Reap S, et al. Transseptal vs trans-apical transcatheter mitral valve-in-valve and valve-in-ring implantation: a systematic review and meta-analysis. Curr Probl Cardiol 2023;48(7):101684.

44. Eleid MF, Wang DD, Pursnani A, et al. 2-year outcomes of transcatheter mitral valve replacement in patients with annular calcification, rings, and bioprostheses. J Am Coll Cardiol 2022;80(23):2171–83.

45. Van MNM, Piazza N, Anderson RH, et al. Anatomy of the mitral valvular complex and its implications for transcatheter interventions for mitral regurgitation. J Am Coll Cardiol 2010;56(8):617–26.

46. Gössl M, Thourani V, Babaliaros V, et al. Early outcomes of transcatheter mitral valve replacement with the Tendyne system in severe mitral annular calcification. EuroIntervention J Eur Collab Work Group Interv Cardiol Eur Soc Cardiol 2022;17(18):1523–31.

47. Beller JP, Rogers JH, Thourani VH, et al. Early clinical results with the Tendyne transcatheter mitral valve replacement system. Ann Cardiothorac Surg 2018;7(6):776–9.

48. Abbott Medical Devices. Clinical Trial to Evaluate the Safety and Effectiveness of Using the Tendyne Transcatheter Mitral Valve System for the Treatment of Symptomatic Mitral Regurgitation. clinicaltrials.gov; 2023 https://clinicaltrials.gov/study/NCT03433274. Accessed July 24, 2023.

49. Makkar R, William O 'Neill, Whisenant B, et al. TCT-8 updated 30-day outcomes for the U.S. early feasibility study of the SAPIEN M3 transcatheter mitral valve replacement System. J Am Coll Cardiol 2019;74(13_Supplement):B8.

50. The ENCIRCLE Trial - Full Text View - ClinicalTrials.gov https://clinicaltrials.gov/ct2/show/NCT04153292. Accessed July 13, 2023.

51. Zahr F, Song HK, Chadderdon SM, et al. 30-day outcomes following transfemoral transseptal transcatheter mitral valve replacement. JACC Cardiovasc Interv 2022;15(1):80–9.

52. Medtronic Cardiovascular. Transcatheter Mitral Valve Replacement With the Medtronic IntrepidTM TMVR System in Patients With Severe Symptomatic Mitral Regurgitation - APOLLO Trial. clinicaltrials.gov; 2023 https://clinicaltrials.gov/study/NCT03242642. Accessed July 24, 2023.

53. Alexis SL, Malik AH, El-Eshmawi A, et al. Surgical and transcatheter mitral valve replacement in mitral annular calcification: a systematic review. J Am Heart Assoc 2021;10(7):e018514.

54. Eleid MF, Cabalka AK, Malouf JF, et al. Techniques and outcomes for the treatment of paravalvular leak. Circ Cardiovasc Interv 2015;8(8):e001945.

55. Al-Hijji MA, El Sabbagh A, Guerrero ME, et al. Paravalvular leak repair after balloon-expandable transcatheter mitral valve implantation in mitral annular calcification: early experience and lessons learned. Cathet Cardiovasc Interv 2019;94(5):764–72.

56. Transcatheter Mitral Valve Replacement: Insights From Early Clinical Experience and Future Challenges | Journal of the American College of Cardiology https://www.jacc.org/doi/full/10.1016/j.jacc.2017.02.045. Accessed July 12, 2023.

57. 1-Year Outcomes of Transcatheter Mitral Valve Replacement in Patients With Severe Mitral Annular Calcification - ClinicalKey https://www.clinicalkey.com/#!/content/playContent/1-s2.0-S0735109718334934?returnurl=https:%2F%2Flinkinghub.elsevier.com%2Fretrieve%2Fpii%2FS0735109718334934%3Fshowall%3Dtrue&referrer=https:%2F%2Fpubmed.ncbi.nlm.nih.gov%2F. Accessed July 27, 2023.

58. Case BC, Lisko JC, Babaliaros VC, et al. LAMPOON techniques to prevent or manage left ventricular outflow tract obstruction in transcatheter mitral valve replacement. Ann Cardiothorac Surg 2021;10(1):172–9.

59. Predictors of Left Ventricular Outflow Tract Obstruction After Transcatheter Mitral Valve Replacement | JACC: Cardiovascular Interventions https://www.jacc.org/doi/abs/10.1016/j.jcin.2018.12.001. Accessed July 27, 2023.

60. Alcohol Septal Ablation to Prevent Left Ventricular Outflow Tract Obstruction During Transcatheter Mitral Valve Replacement - ClinicalKey https://www.clinicalkey.com/#!/content/playContent/1-s2.0-S1936879819305850?returnurl=https:%2F%2Flinkinghub.elsevier.com%2Fretrieve%2Fpii%2FS1936879819305850%3Fshowall%3Dtrue&referrer=https:%2F%2Fpubmed.ncbi.nlm.nih.gov%2F. Accessed July 27, 2023.

61. Short-term results of alcohol septal ablation as a bail-out strategy to treat severe left ventricular outflow tract obstruction after transcatheter mitral valve replacement in patients with severe mitral annular calcification - Guerrero - 2017 - Catheterization and Cardiovascular Interventions - Wiley Online Library https://onlinelibrary.wiley.com/doi/abs/10.1002/ccd.26975. Accessed July 13, 2023.

62. Khan JM, Bruce CG, Greenbaum AB, et al. Transcatheter myotomy to relieve left ventricular outflow tract obstruction: the septal scoring along the midline endocardium procedure in animals. Circ Cardiovasc Interv 2022;15(6):e011686.

63. Greenbaum AB, Khan JM, Bruce CG, et al. Transcatheter myotomy to treat hypertrophic cardiomyopathy and enable transcatheter mitral valve replacement; first-in-human report of SESAME (SEptal Scoring Along the Midline Endocardium). Circ Cardiovasc Interv 2022;15(6):e012106.

Transcatheter Mitral Annuloplasty: Carillon Device

Vinayak Nagaraja, MBBS, MS, MMed (Clin Epi), FRACP[a], Samir R. Kapadia, MD[b],*

KEYWORDS

• Functional mitral regurgitation • Carillon • Mitral annuloplasty

---

KEY POINTS

- Functional mitral regurgitation (FMR) is common in the geriatric population and this cohort commonly has prohibitive risk for cardiac surgery. FMR's anatomical pathology is heterogeneous and one size does not fit all.
- Carillon Mitral Contour System (Cardiac Dimensions, Kirkland, WA, USA) offers transcatheter annular remodeling and studies so far demonstrate consistent reverse remodeling of the left ventricle.
- The Empower study (NCT03142152) we add further to the existing literature.
- Different sequences of percutaneous mitral technologies like indirect annuloplasty and edge-to-edge mitral valve repair need further dedicated clinical trials.
- Further research is essentially addressing to refine the patient selection for this technology by employing Cardiac Computed tomography(CCT) guided Carillon implantation.

INTRODUCTION

The prevalence of mitral regurgitation is nearly 2% in the first world which increases to over 10% in the geriatric population.[1] Functional mitral regurgitation (FMR) due to left ventricular (LV) dysfunction is present in nearly half of the heart failure cohort and prevalent in 25% of the individuals following myocardial infarction.[2] Guideline-directed medical therapy is the cornerstone in the management of FMR; however, a large proportion continues to be symptomatic despite optimal medical therapy.[3] The role of surgery in the form of mitral valve replacement or repair is a suboptimal strategy in this high-risk multimorbid cohort of patients.[4] The COAPT trial was a practice-changing trial in this landscape and the results at 5 years continue to be encouraging.[5] FMR anatomically can be very heterogenous and transcatheter edge-to-edge repair (TEER) may not be feasible or ideal for some individuals.[6] The Carillon Mitral Contour System (Cardiac Dimensions, Kirkland, WA, USA) is a promising new technology that offers transcatheter annular remodeling (TAR) and complements TEER in treating FMR. This article reviews the design, periprocedural planning, and evidence base for the Carillon Mitral Contour System.

ANATOMIC PATHOLOGY OF FUNCTIONAL MITRAL REGURGITATION

The etiology behind FMR is valve malcoaptation primarily due to LV dilatation that results in mitral annular dilatation, apical displacement, and tethering of the mitral leaflets.[7,8] On the other hand, atrial FMR is related to left atrial enlargement due to atrial fibrillation in isolation or in conjunction with heart failure resulting in mitral annular dilatation.[8] These processes result in the reduction of coaptation surface.[9]

Funding: Nil.
[a] Department of Cardiovascular Diseases, Mayo Clinic College of Medicine, Rochester, MN, USA; [b] Department of Cardiovascular Medicine, Cleveland Clinic Foundation, 9500 Euclid Avenue, Cleveland, OH, USA
* Corresponding author.
E-mail address: kapadis@ccf.org

As annular dilation plays a significant role in FMR, anatomic solutions to reduce annular size led to investigating a role for the coronary sinus (CS). The CS is formed by the great cardiac vein and the main posterior lateral vein at the lateral aspect of the LV. The CS runs in the left atrioventricular groove almost parallel to the mitral valve annulus. The CS receives drainage from various tributaries finally draining into the right atrium. The left circumflex artery intersects the CS in 80% of the individuals and the site of intersection ranges between 37 to 123 mm from the CS ostium.[10] The distance between the CS and mitral valve annulus increases in FMR. This is associated with the transformation of the mitral valve annulus with the "flattening" of the conventional saddle-shaped morphology.

DESIGN AND DEPLOYMENT

The Carillon device consists of a nitinol band with 2 self-expanding anchors on either side and is implanted via the right internal jugular vein through a 9 Fr sheath. The distal self-expanding anchor is inserted through the CS and placed before the anterior interventricular vein; later the device is cinched to approximate the annulus. Acute reduction in mitral regurgitation (MR) is not the primary procedural endpoint. After the cinching the annulus, the proximal self-expanding anchor is released, and invasive coronary angiography is performed to assess left circumflex artery extrinsic compression. If there is evidence of left circumflex artery extrinsic compression, adjustments can be made prior to the final release of the Carillon system.

CARDIAC COMPUTED TOMOGRAPHY ANALYSIS

Cardiac computed tomography (CCT) is an essential imaging modality in structural heart intervention.[11,12] All patients undergoing percutaneous indirect mitral annuloplasty should undergo a CCT for procedural planning. A retrospective analysis from Germany assessed 30 patients with preprocedural CCTs and subsequent Carillon device implantation.[13] Based on the 3-month transthoracic echocardiographic follow-up, patients were classified into responders and nonresponders. Using the CCT, the CS and the mitral valve annulus plane were delineated. Later the angle and distance between the 2 planes were analyzed. Based on the analysis, a favorable distance was less than 7.8 mm. The optimal angle was less than 14.2° which had a sensitivity of 87.5% and a specificity

of 100% with a concordance statistic of 96.7%. Another analysis from the same group evaluated the role of CCT in predicting left circumflex compromise.[14] This cohort consisted of 14 patients with left circumflex occlusion/compression and 11 without left circumflex compromise. The CS to left circumflex artery distance of less than 8.6 mm (sensitivity and specificity = 91.7%) in the distal device landing zone was predictive of left circumflex artery compromise. **Fig. 1** demonstrates the reconstruction of different planes to identify high-risk anatomy.

SUMMARY OF THE CLINICAL EVIDENCE

The Carillon Mitral Annuloplasty Device European Union Study (AMADEUS) enrolled 48 patients with moderate to severe FMR, New York Heart Association (NYHA) class III symptoms, and an ejection fraction of less than 40% (dilated cardiomyopathy with a 6-min walk distance(6MWD) ranged from 150 m to 450 m).[15] Only 30 patients underwent successful device implantation and the remaining 18 patients did not undergo device implantation for several reasons. The reasons for device deferral include access site concerns in 5 patients. The device was recaptured for various reasons such as distal anchor slippage (3 patients), insufficient change in FMR after implantation (4 patients), coronary compromise (1 patient), and lastly, the combined insufficient change in FMR after implantation with coronary compromise (5 patients). The patients who underwent device implantation had a mean age of 64 years (standard deviation (SD) ±9 years) and were comprised of mostly men (87%). The mean LV ejection fraction (LVEF) was 30% and most patients (73%) had NYHA class III symptoms. Three individuals developed serum creatine kinase myocardial band elevation with 1 mortality related to multiorgan failure. There were 3 patients who suffered CS dissection or perforation. None of the cohorts needed percutaneous coronary intervention or surgery after device implantation. At 6 months, the FMR improved and the FMR reduction ranged between 22% and 32%. The mean 6MWD improved by nearly 100 m and the mean quality of life (QoL) score based on the Kansas City Cardiomyopathy Questionnaire (KCCQ) improved by 22 points.

The TITAN Trial included 53 patients on optimal medical therapy with at least moderate (2+) FMR, a LVEF of less than 40%, NYHA class II to IV, and 6MWD 150 to 450 m.[16] Patients with severe tricuspid regurgitation, serum creatinine greater than 2.2 mg/dL, and individuals needing

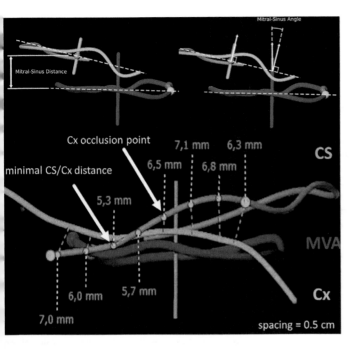

Cx occlusion point   7,1 mm   6,3 mm

minimal CS/Cx distance   6,5 mm   6,8 mm   CS

5,3 mm

MVA

6,0 mm   5,7 mm   Cx

7,0 mm

spacing = 0.5 cm

Mitral-Sinus Angle

Mitral-Sinus Distance

Fig. 1. Cardiac analysis and preprocedural planning for the Carillon device (permission acquired).[13,14] The relationship between the mitral valve annular (MVA: *red*) and the coronary sinus (CS) plane (*blue*) is outlined. Later, the distance and angle between the planes are measured as shown in the top panels. The minimal distance between the coronary sinus plane (*blue*) and the left circumflex (Cx) artery (*green*) is measured as shown in the lower panel.

inotropes in the last 1 month were excluded. The patients were followed for 24 months. Out of the 53 patients, only 36 patients underwent permanent device implantation, mostly men with an average age of just over 62 years, and the mean LVEF was 28%. The remaining 17 patients did not undergo device implantation due to insufficient FMR reduction or coronary compromise. After 12 months of device implantation, there was a significant reduction in the septal-lateral annular diameter, reduction in regurgitant volume, effective regurgitant orifice area, vena contracta, mitral regurgitation jet area/left atrial area, LV end-diastolic diameter (LVEDD)/end-systolic diameter, and volume. At 2 years, there was a significant functional improvement seen in 6MWD and QoL. At 1 year, 8 patients died from a wide range of etiologies. Nine patients experienced a fracture of the anchor wire in the TITAN II trial with the Carillon XE2 device (7 at the proximal end and 2 at the distal end).[16]

The TITAN II trial was the third study to assess the Carillon device.[17] A modified XE2 device was used in the TITAN II trial to address the anchor wire fractures.[17] These modifications include the absence of 'ski slopes' adjacent to either end of the XE2 device and the presence of space between the crimping tube of the proximal anchor and locking loop. In the TITAN II trial, 30 patients underwent device implantation, and 6 individuals experienced coronary compromise; hence, the device was recaptured.[17] The TITAN

II cohort was older (mean age of 70 years) compared to the previous 2 Carillon studies.[15,16] The inclusion and exclusion criteria were congruent to the TITAN trial.[16] The one-year mortality rate for the cohort was 23% with substantial improvement in quantitative parameters of FMR, mitral annular dimensions, NYHA classification, and 6MWD. There were neither device-related major adverse events nor fatigue-related fractures.

The REDUCE FMR trial was the first randomized sham-controlled study evaluating the Carillon device.[18] The trial included overall 120 patients who were enrolled at 24 centers across Europe and Australia (treatment arm 87 patients and sham-controlled arm 33 patients). The primary efficacy endpoint was defined as the change in mitral regurgitant volume at 12 months compared to baseline, and the secondary endpoint consisted of major adverse events that were defined as death, myocardial infarction, device embolization, vessel erosion, cardiac perforation, need for cardiac surgery or percutaneous coronary intervention associated with device failure, and heart failure hospitalizations. The secondary efficacy endpoints constituted changes in LV end-diastolic volume (LVEDV) and LV end-systolic volume (LVESV); changes in 6MWD, NYHA functional class, and QoL at 12 months were compared to baseline. The mean age and LVEF of the treatment arm were 70 years. In the treatment arm of 87 patients, only 73 underwent successful device implantation. The reasons for device retrieval include coronary compromise (8 patients), CS dissection (2 patients), and logistical issues. There were no insistences of device fracture/embolization, cardiac perforations, or intraprocedural myocardial infarctions. At 1 month, there were 2 mortalities, both as a result of worsening cardiorenal syndrome, and 3 myocardial infarctions (1 instance of left circumflex compression). The point estimate for the primary efficacy endpoint was statistically significant (10.39, 95% confidence interval [CI]: 0.06–20.71, P value: 0.049), and there was significant improvement in FMR severity at 1 year. Cardiac resynchronization therapy was possible despite the Carillon device implantation. There was strong evidence to support reverse remodeling with statistically significant reduction in LVEDV (P value = .03) and LVESV (P value = .04) at 1 year. Functional outcomes (6MWD, KCCQ score, and NYHA class) at 12 months were observed to have a tendency toward improvement.[19]

Multiple papers have been published to assess the collective impact of the Carillon device from the REDUCE-FMR, TITAN, and TITAN II studies.[20–23] At 12 months, all mitral valve indices significantly decreased, like mitral regurgitant volume (−12 mL, P value < .001), MR grade (−0.6 U, P value < .001), LVEDV(−25 cm^3, P value = .005), and LVESV (−21 cm^3, P=.01) (Fig. 2). The Carillon device at 12 months significantly improved the 6MWD (64.1 m; 95% CI 13.2–115.0, P=.01), KCCQ score (12.3 points; 95% CI 4.7–19.8, P=.002), and NYHA class (48.8%; 95% CI 31.8–66.2).[21] Long-term data

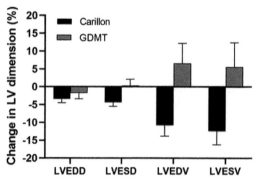

Fig. 2. Pooled analysis of TITAN, TITAN II, and REDUCE FMR trials: Left ventricular (LV) reverse remodeling at 1 year. GDMT, guideline-directed medical therapy; LV, left ventricular; LVEDD, left ventricular end-diastolic diameter; LVEDV, left ventricular end-diastolic volume; LVESD, left ventricular end-systolic diameter; LVESV, left ventricular end-systolic volume. (Permission acquired).[20]

from the REDUCE-FMR, TITAN, and TITAN II studies suggest a favorable 5-year survival rate of 56.2% with the Carillon device.[24] The independent predictors of long-term survival were reduction in NYHA class, an increase in 6MWD, and a reduction in mitral regurgitant volume observed at 12 months of follow-up.[24]

The interim results from CINCH-FMR (NCT05677568) registry was presented at the Transcatheter Cardiovascular Therapeutics conference 2022.[25] The results from 101 patients were presented who had a mean age of 75 years and a mean LVEF of 43%. There were only 2 device-related or procedure-related serious adverse events reported, namely an access site arteriovenous fistula and a pseudoaneurysm. All serious adverse effects amounted to 46.5% at 12 months. The 5-year survival rate was around 56%, similar to the pooled analysis of previous trials.[24] There was significant improvement in NYHA class and FMR reduction at 5 years. Outside of these trials, there have been a couple of small single-center publications with similar results.[26,27]

EDGE-TO-EDGE MITRAL VALVE REPAIR VERSUS INDIRECT ANNULOPLASTY FOR ATRIAL FUNCTIONAL MITRAL REGURGITATION

A retrospective single-center analysis of 41 patients with atrial FMR compared edge-to-edge mitral valve repair (20 patients with MitraClip, Abbott Vascular) to indirect annuloplasty (21 patients with Carillon device).[28] At 1-year follow-up, edge-to-edge repair was better than indirect annuloplasty with regard to reduction in vena contracta (MitraClip −50.8 ± 27.9 vs Carillon −23.9 ± 17.0%, P<.05) and qualitative mitral valve assessment. However, the reduction in left atrial volume at 12 months was superior with post-indirect annuloplasty compared to edge-to-edge repair (MitraClip +9.6 ± 25.1% vs Carillon: vs −12.3 ± 12.7%, P<.05).

FUTURE CARILLON TRIALS

The coronavirus disease 2019 pandemic disrupted the AFIRE (An Initial Evaluation of the Carillon Mitral Contour System for Treatment of Atrial Function Mitral Regurgitation, NCT04529928) and the EXERCISE FMR (Carillon Mitral Contour System for Treatment of Exercise Induced Functional Mitral Regurgitation, NCT05040451) trials. The main reasons for their termination include the inability to recruit patients in the trial and limited hospital resources/staff during the pandemic.

THE EMPOWER TRIAL

The Empower study (NCT03142152) is a prospective randomized, double-blind, sham-controlled international trial being conducted across 3 continents (75 sites) comparing Carillon Mitral Contour System to guideline-directed medical therapy. The trial plans to enroll 300 individuals with a diagnosis of ischemic or nonischemic cardiomyopathy (NYHA class II–IV, LVEF ≤ 50%, LVEDD 60–70 mm) and symptomatic FMR of at least 1+ (mild) severity currently on guideline-directed medical therapy resulting in ≥ 1 heart failure hospitalizations within 6 months or elevated brain natriuretic peptide. The exclusion criteria for this trial include previous cardiac resynchronization therapy or candidates with class I indication for cardiac resynchronization therapy, patients with previous mitral valve repair or replacement, significant mitral valve pathology, severe tricuspid regurgitation with concomitant right ventricular dysfunction, left atrial appendage device or thrombus, severe aortic stenosis/severe mitral annular calcification/severe coronary disease, and a life expectancy of less than 12 months. The primary safety objective includes freedom from a composite of major adverse events like device embolization, cardiac perforation, vessel erosion, and the need for cardiac surgery or percutaneous coronary intervention. The primary efficacy consists of hierarchical clinical composite of heart failure hospitalization, percutaneous or surgical mitral valve intervention, transplant or LV assist device, and death at 1 year. The secondary outcomes include change in LVEDV/LVESV, 6MWD, regurgitant volume, NYHA classification, KCCQ at 1 year. Other secondary outcomes include freedom from a composite of major adverse events like device embolization, cardiac perforation, vessel erosion, and the need for cardiac surgery or percutaneous coronary intervention. The trial is currently recruiting, and the estimated study completion date is December 31, 2028.

SUMMARY

The evidence so far regarding the Carillon device is promising. Reverse LV remodeling after the Carillon implantation has been consistently reproduced across multiple studies.[15–18,23,28,29] Future research is necessary to refine the patient selection for this technology further by employing CCT-guided Carillon implantation. Combination of different percutaneous technologies like indirect annuloplasty and edge-to-edge mitral valve repair, either sequential or concomitant, should be evaluated in future trials. So far, there is only 1 case report published in the literature depicting the initial use of edge-to-edge mitral valve repair followed by indirect annuloplasty 15 months later.[30] The future of FMR intervention is certainly bright, and future trials will make this arena more inclusive for the heterogenous FMR population.

CLINICS CARE POINTS

- Procedural deployment of the Carillon system is relatively straight forward.
- The maximum amount of synching is performed without compromising coronaries, and invasive coronary angiography is performed to assess left circumflex artery extrinsic compression.
- Preprocedural CCT is essential in identifying high-risk features that contribute to left circumflex artery compromise and non responders.
- To identify responders, the coronary sinus and the mitral valve annular planes are defined on CCT. Patients are more likely to respond after deployment, if the optimal angle between the two planes was less than 14.2 degrees and the distance between the two planes was be less than 7.8 mm.
- The coronary sinus to left circumflex artery distance of less than 8.6 mm in the distal device landing zone is predictive of left circumflex artery compromise.

ACKNOWLEDGMENTS

Nil.

DISCLOSURES

No conflict of interest.

REFERENCES

1. d'Arcy JL, Coffey S, Loudon MA, et al. Large-scale community echocardiographic screening reveals a major burden of undiagnosed valvular heart disease in older people: the OxVALVE Population Cohort Study. Eur Heart J 2016;37(47):3515–22.
2. Levine RA, Schwammenthal E. Ischemic mitral regurgitation on the threshold of a solution: from paradoxes to unifying concepts. Circulation 2005; 112(5):745–58.

3. Nishimura RA, Otto CM, Bonow RO, et al. AHA/ACC Focused Update of the 2014 AHA/ACC Guideline for the Management of Patients With Valvular Heart Disease: A Report of the American College of Cardiology/American Heart Association Task Force on Clinical Practice Guidelines. Circulation 2017;135(25):e1159–95.

4. Mihaljevic T, Lam BK, Rajeswaran J, et al. Impact of mitral valve annuloplasty combined with revascularization in patients with functional ischemic mitral regurgitation. J Am Coll Cardiol 2007;49(22):2191–201.

5. Stone GW, Abraham WT, Lindenfeld J, et al. Five-Year Follow-up after Transcatheter Repair of Secondary Mitral Regurgitation. N Engl J Med 2023;388(22):2037–48.

6. Attizzani GF, Ohno Y, Capodanno D, et al. Extended use of percutaneous edge-to-edge mitral valve repair beyond EVEREST (Endovascular Valve Edge-to-Edge Repair) criteria: 30-day and 12-month clinical and echocardiographic outcomes from the GRASP (Getting Reduction of Mitral Insufficiency by Percutaneous Clip Implantation) registry. JACC Cardiovasc Interv 2015;8(1 Pt A):74–82.

7. Chehab O, Roberts-Thomson R, Ng Yin Ling C, et al. Secondary mitral regurgitation: pathophysiology, proportionality and prognosis. Heart 2020;106(10):716–23.

8. Deferm S, Bertrand PB, Verbrugge FH, et al. Atrial Functional Mitral Regurgitation: JACC Review Topic of the Week. J Am Coll Cardiol 2019;73(19):2465–76.

9. Silbiger JJ. Mechanistic insights into atrial functional mitral regurgitation: Far more complicated than just left atrial remodeling. Echocardiography 2019;36(1):164–9.

10. Choure AJ, Garcia MJ, Hesse B, et al. In vivo analysis of the anatomical relationship of coronary sinus to mitral annulus and left circumflex coronary artery using cardiac multidetector computed tomography: implications for percutaneous coronary sinus mitral annuloplasty. J Am Coll Cardiol 2006;48(10):1938–45.

11. Yoon SH, Bleiziffer S, Latib A, et al. Predictors of Left Ventricular Outflow Tract Obstruction After Transcatheter Mitral Valve Replacement. JACC Cardiovasc Interv 2019;12(2):182–93.

12. Francone M, Budde RPJ, Bremerich J, et al. CT and MR imaging prior to transcatheter aortic valve implantation: standardisation of scanning protocols, measurements and reporting-a consensus document by the European Society of Cardiovascular Radiology (ESCR). Eur Radiol 2020;30(5):2627–50.

13. Rottländer D, Ballof J, Gödde M, et al. CT-Angiography to predict outcome after indirect mitral annuloplasty in patients with functional mitral regurgitation. Catheter Cardiovasc Interv 2021;97(3):495–502.

14. Rottländer D, Gödde M, Degen H, et al. Procedural planning of CS-based indirect mitral annuloplasty using CT-angiography. Catheter Cardiovasc Interv 2021;98(7):1393–401.

15. Schofer J, Siminiak T, Haude M, et al. Percutaneous mitral annuloplasty for functional mitral regurgitation: results of the CARILLON Mitral Annuloplasty Device European Union Study. Circulation 2009;120(4):326–33.

16. Siminiak T, Wu JC, Haude M, et al. Treatment of functional mitral regurgitation by percutaneous annuloplasty: results of the TITAN Trial. Eur J Heart Fail 2012;14(8):931–8.

17. Lipiecki J, Siminiak T, Sievert H, et al. Coronary sinus-based percutaneous annuloplasty as treatment for functional mitral regurgitation: the TITAN II trial. Open Heart 2016;3(2):e000411.

18. Witte KK, Lipiecki J, Siminiak T, et al. The REDUCE FMR Trial: A Randomized Sham-Controlled Study of Percutaneous Mitral Annuloplasty in Functional Mitral Regurgitation. JACC Heart Fail 2019;7(11):945–55.

19. Khan MS, Siddiqi TJ, Butler J, et al. Functional outcomes with Carillon device over 1 year in patients with functional mitral regurgitation of Grades 2+ to 4+: results from the REDUCE-FMR trial. ESC Heart Fail 2021;8(2):872–8.

20. Anker SD, Starling RC, Khan MS, et al. Percutaneous Mitral Valve Annuloplasty in Patients With Secondary Mitral Regurgitation and Severe Left Ventricular Enlargement. JACC Heart Fail 2021;9(6):453–62.

21. Khan MS, Friede T, Anker SD, et al. Effect of Carillon Mitral Contour System on patient-reported outcomes in functional mitral regurgitation: an individual participant data meta-analysis. ESC Heart Fail 2021;8(3):1885–91.

22. Giallauria F, Di Lorenzo A, Parlato A, et al. Individual patient data meta-analysis of the effects of the CARILLON® mitral contour system. ESC Heart Fail 2020;7(6):3383–91.

23. Witte KK, Kaye DM, Lipiecki J, et al. Treating symptoms and reversing remodelling: clinical and echocardiographic 1-year outcomes with percutaneous mitral annuloplasty for mild to moderate secondary mitral regurgitation. Eur J Heart Fail 2021;23(11):1971–8.

24. Lipiecki J, Kaye DM, Witte KK, et al. Long-term survival following transcatheter mitral valve repair: Pooled analysis of prospective trials with the Carillon device. Cardiovasc Revascularization Med 2020;21(20):30082–8.

25. Witte K, Haude M, Goldberg S. TCT-416 Interim Results of the CINCH-FMR Post-Market Registry: Percutaneous Repair in Functional Mitral

Regurgitation (FMR) With the Carillon Mitral Contour System. J Am Coll Cardiol 2022;80(12_Supplement):B168–.

26. Kałmucki P, Jerzykowska O, Dankowski R, et al. Percutaneous Trans-Coronary Venous Mitral Annuloplasty in Patients With Functional Mitral Regurgitation: Analysis of Poznan Carillon Registry Data. J Interv Cardiol 2016;29(6):632–8.

27. Lipiecki J, Fahrat H, Monzy S, et al. Long-term prognosis of patients treated by coronary sinus-based percutaneous annuloplasty: single centre experience. ESC Heart Fail 2020;7(6):3329–35.

28. Rottländer D, Golabkesh M, Degen H, et al. Mitral valve edge-to-edge repair versus indirect mitral valve annuloplasty in atrial functional mitral regurgitation. Catheter Cardiovasc Interv 2022;99(6):1839–47.

29. Ruf TF, Kreidel F, Tamm AR, et al. Transcatheter indirect mitral annuloplasty induces annular and left atrial remodelling in secondary mitral regurgitation. ESC Heart Fail 2020;7(4):1400–8.

30. Abdelrahman N, Chowdhury MA, Al Nooryani A, et al. A case of dilated cardiomyopathy and severe mitral regurgitation treated using a combined percutaneous approach of MitraClip followed by CARILLON® mitral contour system. Cardiovasc Revascularization Med 2016;17(8):578–81.

Minimally Invasive Mitral Valve Repair Using Transcatheter Chordal Attachments

Chandan Das, MD[a], Ghayth Al Awwa, MBBS[a],
Emmanuel L. Mills, MD[b], Gurion Lantz, MD[a],*

KEYWORDS

- Mitral valve • Transcatheter mitral valve interventions
- Transcatheter mitral neochordal replacement

KEY POINTS

- Transcatheter chordal replacement options are being heavily investigated with several exciting new devices in the pipeline.
- Isolated prolapsed segments, especially central segments, are the most amenable to transcatheter or transapical chordal replacement therapy.
- Percutaneous transcatheter devices are earlier in their development than transapical devices, but because of the requirement for surgery for transapical access, the transapical devices have not yet been widely adopted.

INTRODUCTION

Mitral valve disease is a globally significant medical challenge, contributing to considerable morbidity and mortality. It is characterized by either mitral stenosis or mitral regurgitation (MR), either of which often culminates in heart failure if left untreated. Mitral stenosis, generally caused by rheumatic heart disease, is typically treated with valve replacement or balloon valvuloplasty. On the other hand, MR has a wider spectrum of causes, including myxomatous degeneration, functional and ischemic MR, rheumatic heart disease, and mitral annular calcification. MR can be approached with either repair or replacement depending on the details of the pathologic condition. Repair techniques for MR include annuloplasty, leaflet resection or augmentation, and chordal replacement.

As medical technology advances, with a growing inclination toward minimally invasive interventions, the landscape of treatments for mitral valve disease has been evolving. One of the most impactful innovations in this realm has been transcatheter edge-to-edge therapy, which has significantly altered the treatment landscape and become a major pillar in the management of MR. Another emerging approach is to use transcatheter chordal replacement (Fig. 1). Designed to replicate the natural chordae tendineae anchoring the mitral valve leaflets, chordal replacements offer a promising, albeit still evolving, alternative for patients who may be at high risk with traditional surgical methods. Overall, transcatheter therapies, whether focused on repair or evolving replacement strategies, are reshaping the approach to mitral valve disease.

This article explores emerging transcatheter chordal replacement techniques in contrast with surgical repair or transcatheter edge-to-edge repair (TEER) techniques. By highlighting the strengths and limitations of each approach,

---

[a] Oregon Health and Science University, 3181 Southwest Sam Jackson Park Road, Mail Code L353, Portland, OR 97239, USA; [b] Knight Cardiovascular Institute, Oregon Health and Science University, 3181 Southwest Sam Jackson Park Road, Mail Code UHN-62, Portland, OR 97239, USA
* Corresponding author.
E-mail address: lantz@ohsu.edu

Intervent Cardiol Clin 13 (2024) 257–269
https://doi.org/10.1016/j.iccl.2023.12.006
2211-7458/24/© 2024 Elsevier Inc. All rights reserved.

Device	Approach	Attachment Modality	Clinical/Preclinical Studies and Approval Status
Neochord DS 1000 (NeoChord, Inc., USA)	Transapical, off-pump beating heart neochordae	Direct leaflet puncutre with PTFE suture and tensioning at PTFE pledget apical epicardial anchor	TACT (early, 1 year, 3 year, and 5 year followup studies), ReChord (RCT)[13,14,15] CE Mark (2012), FDA IDE (2016)
Harpoon TDS-5 (Edwards Lifesciences, USA)	Transapical, off pump neochordae tensioned in real-time	PTFE apical pledge/ pre-knotted PTFE suture, suture passer system for leaflet puncture	TRACER (6 month followup), REPLICATE (1 year followup study - terminated for low enrollment), RESTORE (prospective, non-randomized trial - terminated)[16,17] CE Mark (2020), FDA IDE (2020), trials and device withdrawn
MitralStitch (Hangzhou DeJin Medtech Co., China)	Transapical, off pump neochordae tensioned in real-time	Pledgeted PTFE suture leaflet anchor and PTFE pledget apical epicardial anchor	Early first-in-man with 1 month and 1 year followup[18,19] CE Mark (study complete, approval pending)
NeoChord NeXuS (NeoChord, Inc.. USA)	Transseptal, off-pump neochordae with RT tensioning	Girth Hitch knot leaflet anchor with nitinol papillary muscle andchor	First-in-man completed[26] Early feasibility trial currently enrolling
CardioMech (CardioMech, AS, Norway)	Transseptal, off-pump neochordae with RT tensioning	Direct suture anchor of leaflet and self-expanding nitinol papillary muscle anchor	First in man study with 3 devices implanted with 100% detachment of papillary anchor[23]
ChordArt (CoreMedic GmbH, Germany)	Transseptal device premeasured neochords	Nitinol leaflet anchor with premeasured chord length and papillary muscle nitinol anchor	First-in-man study completed with 2 year followup[25] CE Mark study planned
Pipeline (Gore, Inc., USA)	Transseptal, off-pump neochordae with premeasured lengths	Nitinol leaflet anchor with PTFE neochord and nitinol ventricular papillary muscle anchor	First-in-man presented at TCT with detachment of leaflet anchor requiring elective surgical intervention the following week[22]
Mitral Butterfly (Angel Valve, Austria)	Transseptal, off-pump leaflet stabilization device and neochord implantation	Nitinol leaflet frame with PET mesh and PTFE neochords without myocardial fixation	Preclinical animal testing
V-Chordal (Valtech, Israel)	Transseptal, off-pump leaflet stabilization device and neochord implantation	Hook needles leaflet anchor with PTFE neochordae and nitinol papillary muscle anchor	Preclinical animal testing

Fig. 1. Comparison of various percutaneous and transapical mitral valve neochordal devices and their current stages of development.

the authors aim to provide an overview of the contemporary strategies for mitral valve repair and patient selection considerations as these treatment modalities evolve.

ANATOMY AND PATHOPHYSIOLOGY

Understanding the complexities of mitral valve disease begins with a deep appreciation of the intricate anatomy of the mitral valve and the pathophysiologic processes that culminate in disease. The mitral valve is one of the 4 valves in the heart, located between the left atrium and left ventricle, playing an essential role in maintaining unidirectional blood flow during the cardiac cycle. The valve comprises 2 leaflets—anterior and posterior—connected to the papillary muscles in the left ventricle via fibrous cords known as the chordae tendineae. The coordinated action of these components during systole and diastole ensures the effective and efficient propulsion of blood from the heart to the systemic circulation.

MR is characterized by the backflow of blood from the left ventricle to the left atrium during systole owing to incomplete closure of the mitral valve. Causes are varied and include structural/ degenerative valve pathologic condition, such as chordal rupture or leaflet prolapse, as well as functional changes owing to left ventricular remodeling or annular dilatation, as seen in conditions like ischemic heart disease.[1]

Degenerative MR is characterized by structural abnormalities of the mitral valve apparatus itself, involving the leaflets or chordae tendineae. Herein lies the particular relevance of transcatheter chordal attachments, designed to mimic the function of native chordae tendineae and restore normal valve function.

Understanding the detailed anatomy of the mitral valve and the pathophysiologic processes underpinning the natural history of mitral valve disease is crucial to appreciate the rationale behind therapeutic interventions. This knowledge forms the basis for the subsequent discussion of surgical techniques and transcatheter interventions in managing mitral valve disease.

SURGICAL MITRAL VALVE REPAIR

Traditional surgical techniques have long been the cornerstone of mitral valve repair. The choice of surgical approach—be it annuloplasty, chordal replacement, or leaflet repair—is dependent on the underlying pathologic condition causing mitral valve disease. A thorough understanding of these techniques is fundamental to appreciating their role in managing mitral valve disease and how they compare with the emerging transcatheter methods.

Annuloplasty

Annuloplasty is a surgical technique used predominantly for treating MR and typically involves fixation of a prosthetic ring to the mitral annulus, the fibrous base to which the mitral leaflets are attached. Over time, the annulus may dilate as the left atrium and/or left ventricle dilate secondary to ischemic heart disease[2] or ongoing MR from degenerative valve disease.[3,4] This dilation often exacerbates improper coaptation of the valve leaflets, resulting in worsened regurgitation.

During annuloplasty, a surgeon implants a prosthetic ring or band around the annulus to restore its normal size and shape. This annuloplasty ring serves to facilitate proper leaflet coaptation and prevent future annular dilatation. Annuloplasty rings come in various sizes and shapes and can be rigid, semirigid, or flexible, with each type providing different degrees of annular stabilization and flexibility.

Chordal Replacement

The chordae tendineae are pivotal in maintaining the structural integrity of the mitral valve, preventing leaflet prolapse into the left atrium during systole. However, mitral valve degeneration can lead to the rupture or elongation of these chords, resulting in MR.

Chordal replacement surgery involves replacing the damaged chordae with prosthetic materials, such as expanded polytetrafluoroethylene (ePTFE) sutures.[5] The surgeon attaches these sutures to the affected leaflet segment and then to the corresponding papillary muscle, mimicking the action of native chordae. The length of the suture is adjusted to ensure optimal leaflet mobility, leaflet coaptation, height, and valve competency, reducing regurgitation.

Leaflet Repair

In cases where the leaflets themselves are damaged, deformed, or redundant, leaflet repair may be necessary. This can involve a variety of techniques, such as leaflet resection, where a portion of a prolapsed leaflet is removed, or leaflet plication, where the leaflet is folded and sutured to reduce the prolapse.

Other less-common methods, like edge-to-edge repair, also known as the Alfieri stitch, involve suturing the middle of the anterior and posterior leaflets together to create a double orifice valve, reducing regurgitation.

These surgical techniques—annuloplasty, chordal replacement,[6] and leaflet repair—have served as the bedrock for the treatment of mitral valve disease.[7] They have proven their efficacy over many years of practice, with long-term follow-up studies demonstrating significant improvements in symptoms, left ventricular function, and patient survival.[8] However, as with all surgical procedures, they are not without risk and are associated with a degree of morbidity and mortality.

TRANSCATHETER MITRAL VALVE REPAIR

The advent of transcatheter mitral repair techniques has offered an alternative approach that is less invasive and may be more suitable for select patients compared with surgical repair. TEER, inspired by the surgical technique of edge-to-edge mitral valve repair, has been shown to be safe and effective in select patients based on the EVEREST II and COAPT trials.[9,10] Although TEER has changed the landscape of MR treatment, edge-to-edge therapy is not suitable for all patients. Anatomic considerations, the extent of calcification, and the complexity of the regurgitation play roles in patient selection. The structure and configuration of the mitral valve apparatus are crucial when considering TEER therapy. Specific criteria must be met for the procedure to be successful. The device needs to securely grasp the leaflets, which might be challenging if there is a broad flail segment or extensive billowing of the leaflets. Sufficient length and depth of mitral leaflet coaptation are required for effective clip placement. Edge-to-edge repair can also worsen preexisting stenosis. Presence of extensive calcification on the leaflet or annulus can also pose technical challenges. Although TEER has been used for both degenerative and functional MR, the pathophysiology differs. Degenerative MR, resulting from structural abnormalities like leaflet prolapse, might be more amenable to TEER compared with functional MR, which arises from ventricular remodeling and dilation. Moreover, regurgitation from the central portion of the valve (A2-P2 segments) is generally more amenable to TEER than MR originating from the lateral or medial commissures. TEER is not always a definitive solution. Although it effectively reduces MR and improves symptoms in many patients, it does not address the root cause of the valve dysfunction in all cases. Therefore, some patients may see a recurrence or persistence of MR or might require additional interventions in the future.

In summary, although TEER is a revolutionary tool in the realm of MR management, its application is tempered by a blend of anatomic, pathophysiologic, and technical factors. A comprehensive evaluation by a multidisciplinary heart team helps to ensure that appropriate patients derive maximum benefit from this innovative therapy.

As technology and techniques continue to evolve, the role of the TEER in managing MR is likely to expand and refine, with ongoing research and trials shaping its future indications and uses.

Following the success and recognition of TEER in managing MR, further device investigations are underway that could address mitral valve pathologic conditions, especially for those cases where edge-to-edge mitral therapy might not be the optimal solution. Although TEER mimics the edge-to-edge surgical technique, transcatheter chordal replacement systems draw inspiration from surgical chordal replacement. These devices are designed to emulate the natural chordae tendineae, fibrous cords that play a crucial role in anchoring the mitral valve leaflets and preventing prolapse. Transcatheter leaflet augmentation strategies seek to treat regurgitation by improving leaflet coaptation with the implantation of additional material.

TRANSCATHETER CHORDAL REPLACEMENT

Transcatheter chordal replacement systems involve introducing artificial chordae, to replace or supplement damaged or elongated natural chordae. These artificial chordae are then anchored at one end to the mitral leaflet and the other end to the myocardium, restoring the leaflet's coaptation and reducing regurgitation. Their potential benefit is providing targeted intervention by addressing specific leaflet prolapse or flail segments. The procedure involves the delivery of artificial chordae, often made from durable materials such as ePTFE, via a transcatheter or transapical approach to the affected mitral leaflet. These artificial chordae are anchored to the ventricular apex or the left ventricular wall and tensioned to correct leaflet prolapse, thereby reducing or eliminating MR. Multiple devices are under investigation, with

varying methods of chordal attachment and delivery systems. The space is divided into devices with transapical delivery systems, including the NeoChord DS1000 device, the Harpoon Mitral Valve Repair System, and the MitralStitch System, and devices that have a completely transcatheter delivery, including the NeoChord NeXuS, CardioMech, and Pipeline devices.

Early trials and studies suggest promising results in terms of safety and efficacy in reducing MR severity and improving symptoms. However, comprehensive long-term data are still to be determined. Selecting the right patients for transcatheter chordal replacement is paramount. Not all MR cases stem from chordal issues, so precise diagnosis and assessment are essential. In addition, although these devices offer a less-invasive alternative, the learning curve for practitioners can be steep, given the procedure's technical aspects.

TRANSCATHETER LEAFLET AUGMENTATION SYSTEMS

Leaflet augmentation is a fairly new strategy in the transcatheter treatment of functional MR, using the addition of prosthetic material to enhance the coaptation of the functioning native leaflet tissue.

Half Moon Device

The Half Moon (Half Moon Medical, Palo Alto, CA, USA) device (Fig. 2) is a transfemoral, fully recoverable coaptation augmentation device that consists of a nitinol ring containing a posterior leaflet baffle and anchoring modalities. When the baffle is deployed, it fills the regurgitant orifice and augments the posterior leaflet, altering the coaptation plane to reduce severity of MR. The device contains a posterior clip near the baffle to provide subannular fixation as well as an atrial brim to anchor the device on the atrial side. First-in-man was performed recently at the authors' institution with excellent results.[11] Thirty-day follow-up TTE showed durable decrease in IIIb functional mitral regurgitation (FMR) from 4+ to trace with no change in implant position, coaptation, or function. Prospective, multicenter, nonrandomized early feasibility study is currently underway.

TRANSAPICAL CHORDAL REPLACEMENT SYSTEMS

Neochord DS1000

The NeoChord (Neochord, St. Louis Park, MN, USA) system (Fig. 3) is primarily aimed at addressing degenerative MR. It involves transapical

A

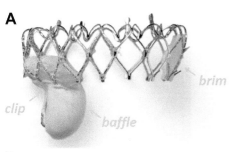

B

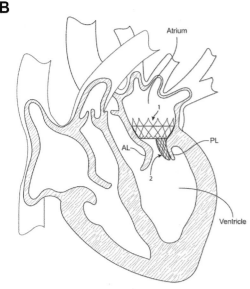

Fig. 2. Half Moon. (A) Half Moon device comprising a nitinol frame with a posterior leaflet clip and baffle as well as an atrial brim that provides attachment at the atrial aspect of the device above the anterior mitral leaflet. (B) Technical drawing from the device patent that shows (1) supra-annular implantation of the device frame with (2) posterior leaflet baffle in place.[11] AL, anterior leaflet; PL, posterior leaflet.

delivery of PTFE suture via a small thoracotomy overlying the apex of the left ventricle. After gaining transapical access, the delivery system crosses the valve and grasps onto the affected leaflet, confirming the correct position by sending information from the jaws via fiberoptic technology to a designated monitor. The delivery system then affixes the neochord system through a leaflet puncture. The chord is thereby secured to the leaflet and then pulled and anchored to the myocardial apex site. The process is performed under real-time transesophageal echocardiographic (TEE) guidance. A key feature of this device is that apical fixation of the device happens after real-time adjustment of the chord length to eliminate regurgitation under TEE guidance.[12]

Positive results from early clinical trials have gathered the device a CE Mark and a Food and Drug Administration (FDA) investigational device exemption. The TACT (Transapical Artificial Chordae Tendinae) trial showed promising results for the NeoChord system, with significant reductions in MR and improvements in patients' symptoms and quality of life.

Gerosa and colleagues[13] reported a 3-year follow-up experience among 200 patients who successfully underwent NeoChord DS1000 placement for severe degenerative MR. Survival and reintervention rates at 3 years were 94.0% and 6.4%, respectively. This suggested that the NeoChord DS1000 system was safe and effective. Through the course of the study, early clinical and echocardiographic data showed not only significant symptomatic relief but also sustained reduction in MR with good left ventricular remodeling and low reintervention rates. The investigators further examined the effect of different anatomic lesions on repair outcomes, with results suggesting that the NeoChord DS1000 system has the best outcomes in patients with posterior leaflet prolapse.

D'Onofrio and colleagues[14] compared outcomes of the NeoChord system versus traditional surgical repair. In a retrospective approach, propensity matching was used to select 88 pairs. Kaplan-Meier analysis showed similar 5-year survival in the 2 groups. However, freedom from recurrent MR was only 57.6% in the NeoChord group and 84.6% in the surgical repair group, and the freedom from reoperation was 78.9% in the NeoChord group and 92% in the surgical group. However, subset analysis in patients with isolated P2 prolapse demonstrated no significant difference in freedom from recurrent MR (63.9% with NeoChord vs 74.6% with open repair) and freedom from reoperation (79.7% with NeoChord vs 85% with open repair). Demonstrating that transapical beating-heart mitral valve chordae implantation can be considered as an alternative treatment for degenerative MR, especially in patients with isolated P2 prolapse.

ReChord (Randomized Trial of the Neochord DS1000 System vs Open Surgical Repair) is a large, randomized, multicenter study that began enrolling in November 2016, with plans for recruiting 585 patients to assess the safety and effectiveness of the device compared with open surgical repair. The study is estimated to be completed by July 2027.[15]

Harpoon TDS-5

The Harpoon (Edwards Lifesciences, Irvine, CA, USA) system uses a handheld delivery system for transapical chordal replacement via a small thoracotomy overlying the apex of the left ventricle. It allows for implantation of multiple and individually adjustable PTFE chordae.

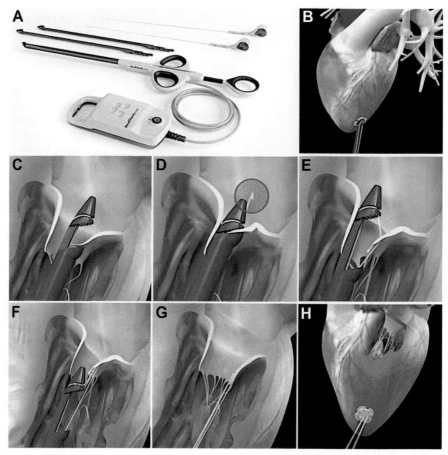

Fig. 3. Neochord DS1000. (*A*) Neochord delivery system. (*B*) Passage of device through LV apex. (2) Grasping of leaflet. (*D*) Leaflet puncture. (*E*) Deployment of leaflet anchor. (*F, G*) Device withdrawal. (*H*) Chordal tensioning and apical anchor deployment. Courtesy of Neochord Inc.

Under TEE guidance, the Harpoon device is inserted and navigated to the prolapsed segment of the posterior leaflet. The leaflet is then punctured, and an ePTFE chord is knotted on the atrial side of the leaflet. The cord is externalized through the introducer, and then real-time tensioning to eliminate regurgitation is performed under TEE guidance. The chordae are then affixed at the apical access site (Fig. 4).

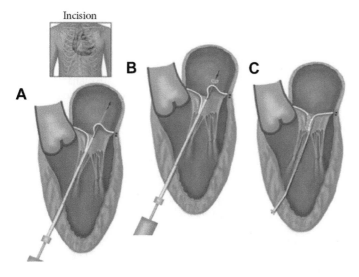

Fig. 4. Harpoon TDS-5. (*A*) Passage of device through LV apex and leaflet puncture. (*B*) Deployment of leaflet anchor. (*C*) Chordal tensioning and apical anchor deployment.[16]

The initial feasibility study for the Harpoon device enrolled 30 patients with severe degenerative MR. At 1 month postprocedure, MR was mild or less in 89% of patients and moderate in 11% of patients. At 6 months, MR was mild or less in 85% of patients, moderate in 8% of patients, and severe in 8% of patients.[16] The same group[17] reported 1-year results of the Harpoon system. Sixty-five patients were enrolled, and 62 (95%) patients achieved procedural success. Two patients required conversion to open surgery, and one patient was terminated from the study. During the perioperative period, the rate of mortality, stroke rate, renal failure, and atrial fibrillation rate were 0%, 0%, 0%, and 18%, respectively. Atrial fibrillation was pooled only for those without baseline atrial fibrillation (n = 50). At 1 year, 2 of the 62 patients died (3%), and 8 (13%) patients required reoperation. At 1 year, 98% of patients with the Harpoon chordae were New York Heart Association functional class I or II, and MR was none to trace in 52%, mild in 23%, moderate in 23%, and severe in 2%. Favorable cardiac remodeling outcomes at 1 year included decreased end-diastolic left ventricular volume and diameter, and a low mean transmitral gradient of 1.4 ± 0.7 mm Hg. This early clinical experience with the Harpoon system demonstrated encouraging early safety and performance; however, the Harpoon system is no longer available for trials or implantation through investigational device exemption (IDE). Long-term data from treated patients may yet be useful for future device design in terms of evaluating the durability of this method of leaflet and apical attachments.

MitralStitch

MitralStitch (Hangzhou DeJin Medtech Co, Hangzhou, China) was the first product to offer both edge-to-edge repair and chordae repair (Fig. 5). In the first-in-human experience, MitralStitch was successfully deployed in 10 patients with severe MR. Nine patients underwent chordal repair alone, and one patient received combined chordal and edge-to-edge repair.[18] At discharge, MR decreased from severe to trace in 5 patients and was mild in the other 5 patients. At 1-year follow-up, 6 patients had mild MR; 3 patients had moderate MR, and one patient had recurrence of severe MR and underwent surgical repair.[19]

TRANSCATHETER CHORDAL REPLACEMENT SYSTEMS

Transcatheter chordal repair devices are attractive because of the minimally invasive nature of

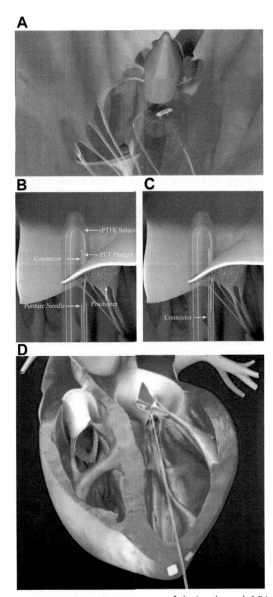

Fig. 5. MitralStitch. (A) Passage of device through MV and alignment using TEE guidance. (B, C) engagement of leaflet positioner and deployment of ePTFE suture and pledget to anchor chord. (D) Real-time chordal tensioning and apical pledgeted securement. ePTFE, expanded polytetrafluoroethylene.

the approach and shorter recovery times than both conventional open repair and transapical repair. However, all of the following products are currently in preclinical stages. The best known devices are the NeoChord NeXuS (NeoChord, USA), ChordArt (CoreMedic, Germany), CardioMech (CardioMech, Norway), Pipeline (Gore, USA). The devices are implanted transseptally through a femoral venous access.

Unlike transapical chordal replacement devices, transcatheter devices require the implantation of metal anchors to hold sutures to the papillary muscle, which carry a small risk of damaging the myocardium of the papillary muscle. Animal studies of the Neochord NeXuS system showed that the anchor nail on the papillary muscle was covered by fibrous tissue and endothelium at 90 days. Overall, the papillary muscle healed well overall, and no obvious necrosis was observed. A study in sheep[20] compared the healing difference between metal screw anchors and surgical sutures anchoring the papillary muscle as in the V-chordal system, and both showed good healing of at 90 days. Animal experiments with the Pipeline system also confirmed that the metal anchors did not damage the papillary muscle. These experiments provided preliminary confirmation of the in vivo safety of metal anchors for anchoring the papillary muscle. In summary, transcatheter chordae repair devices are still in the early stages of development owing to their technical complexity, and only a few clinical trials have been reported.

Gore Pipeline

The Pipeline system (Fig. 6) is a transfemoral, transvenous neochordal device using a ventricular neopapillary anchor and up to 3 pledgeted sutures per anchor. After fixation on the mitral leaflet, the sutures are tensioned under real-time echocardiographic guidance and are then locked in place.[21] Rogers and colleagues[22] reported the first-in-man deployment of the Pipeline system in a 56-year-old male patient with severe MR owing to prolapse in the P2 region. Two artificial chordae were successfully implanted transeptally and attached to a papillary muscle base anchor, eliminating MR intraoperatively. However, the papillary muscle anchor was found to be dislodged before discharge, resulting in recurrent MR, and the patient ultimately underwent mitral valve replacement. The investigators concluded that the ventricular anchor displacement was related to a device technical issue and have reopened the clinical trial after device redesign.

CardioMech

The CardioMech (CardioMech, AS, Trondheim, Norway) system (Fig. 7) uses a single chord with metal anchors on either end that attach to the leaflet and to the left ventricular free wall. The system is tensioned in real-time under TEE guidance. The anchors can be repositioned, which allows for a late point of no return. Rinaldi[23] reported a trial of the CardioMech system in 3 patients with P2 prolapse. Inclusion criteria included patients that were at intermediate to high risk for surgery. MR was reduced from severe to mild or less after successful implantation of one chord, with no serious adverse events occurring during the procedures. However, postoperative dislodgement of the leaflet anchor nail occurred in all 3 patients, and the study was ultimately unsuccessful. CardioMech is in the process of redesigning their device considering these results.

ChordArt

The ChordArt (CoreMedic GmbH, Radolfzell, Germany) device (Fig. 8) is a transfemoral, transseptal device currently in development.[24] Uniquely, the company obtained a CE Mark on the chordal system and opted to implant surgically through standard median sternotomy on cardiopulmonary bypass combined with standard surgical ring annuloplasty in all patients. This has yielded positive 2-year data on the efficacy of the system[25] in a study of 5 patients. All

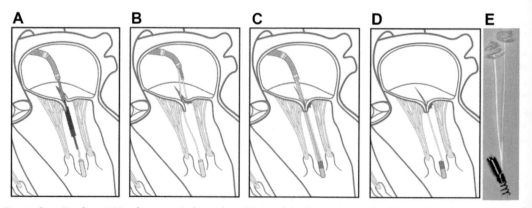

Fig. 6. Gore Pipeline. (A) Implant ventricular anchor. (B) Attach leaflet anchors. (C) Adjust and lock sutures with TTE guidance. (D) Fully deployed. (E) Depiction of the Pipeline device.[21]

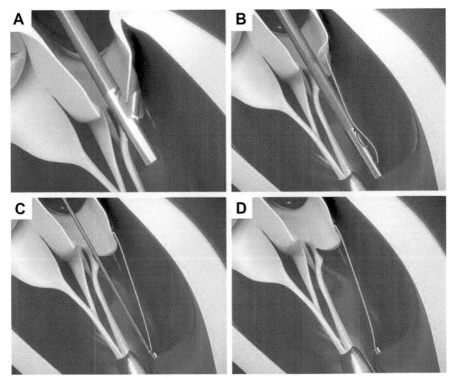

Fig. 7. CardioMech. (A) Leaflet capture and chordal attachment. (B) Positioning ventricular anchor. (C) Ventricular anchor placed. (D) Final after chordal tensioning and anchor deployment.[23]

of the patients postoperatively had trace MR or less, and over 24 months, MR < 1+ was maintained. The company is continuing development of the transseptal delivery system and plans a 40-patient trial that is expected to start recruiting soon. The disadvantage of the system is that the implants have to be premeasured, which precludes beating-heart tensioning.

Neochord NeXuS

The Neochord NeXuS (NeoChord, Inc, St. Louis Park, MN, USA) is a transfemoral,

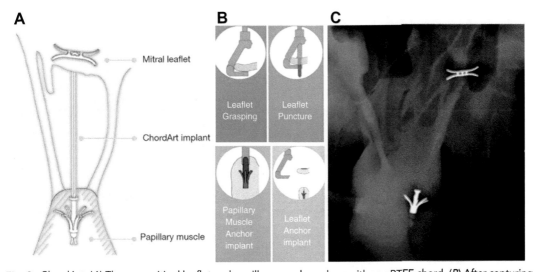

Fig. 8. ChordArt. (A) There are nitinol leaflet and papillary muscle anchors with an ePTFE chord. (B) After capturing the prolapsing segment, a single needle is advanced through the leaflet and into the papillary muscle. The papillary muscle anchor is deployed by retraction of the needle, and then the leaflet anchor is deployed before withdrawal of the device. (C) Postdeployment fluoroscopy.[24]

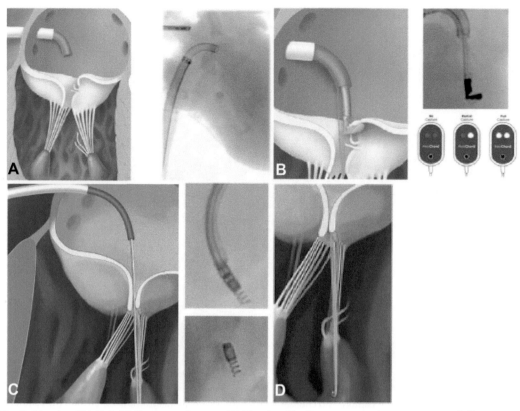

Fig. 9. Neochord NeXuS. (A) Transseptal access. (B) Neochord leaflet capture and engagement with fluoroscopic guidance and sensor confirmation. (C) Passage of device into papillary muscle and deployment of anchor. (D) Final result.[26]

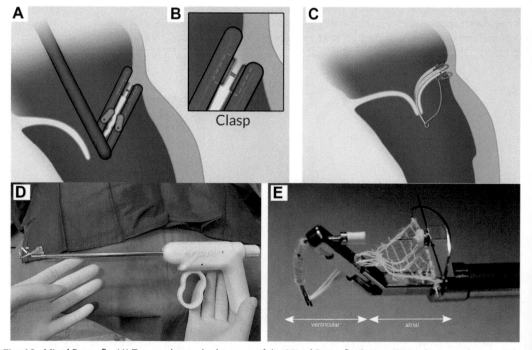

Fig. 10. Mitral Butterfly. (A) Transcatheter deployment of the Mitral Butterfly device. (B) Implant attachment with a single clasp in the periannular region. (C) Deployed Mitral Butterfly device restoring a normal coaptation plane. (D) 24-French transatrial delivery system. (E) Upper (atrial wing and polymer mesh) and lower (swing arm) parts of the implant. The upper (atrial) arm is placed above the leaflet, and the lower (ventricular) arm is wedged underneath the leaflet during device placement.[27]

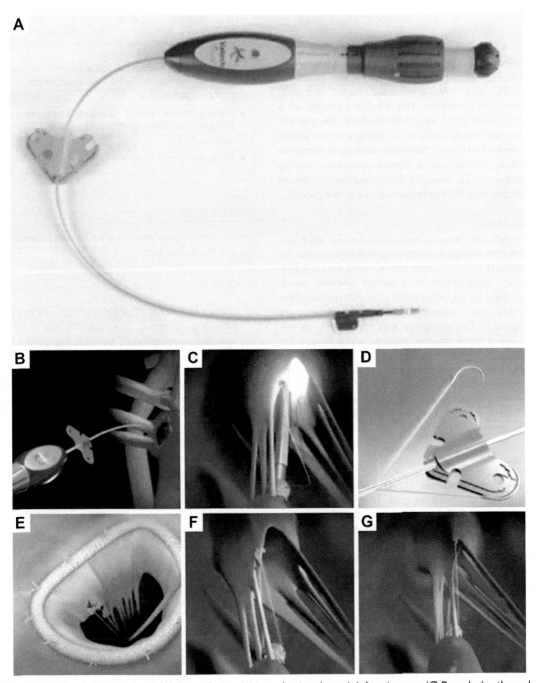

Fig. 11. V-Chordal. (A) V-Chordal delivery device. (B) Introduction through left atriotomy. (C) Pass device through mitral valve and deploy ventricular anchor. (D) Release leaflet sutures. (E) Pass leaflet sutures through leaflet. (F) Tension neochords and attach to leaflet. (G) Fully deployed neochord.[28]

transseptal device based on the transapical Neochord DS1000 platform (Fig. 9). The mitral leaflet is captured under TEE guidance, and placement is confirmed by a fiberoptic sensor. Multiple chordae are attached to a papillary muscle metal screw anchor. Recently, the

first-in-human trial implanted the Neochord NeXuS in 3 patients and reported 6-month follow-up results.[26] The device implantation successfully reduced MR and maintained mild or trace MR at 6 months without displacement of anchors.

PRECLINICAL SYSTEMS

Mitral Butterfly

The Mitral Butterfly system (Fig. 10) is a chordal mesh repair system developed by Angel Valve (Vienna, Austria). It attaches to the posterior leaflet, and with a chordal mesh, prevents continued prolapse. The device consists of a PTFE mesh atrial wing that stabilizes the implant in the left atrium and a nitinol swing arm that allows unrestricted flow in diastole and restricts motion in systole, mimicking a chordal/papillary muscle complex.[27] To date, the device has demonstrated efficacy with 90-day follow-up in a swine model.

V-Chordal

Valtech (Or Yehuda, Israel) has developed a system that allows for on-pump delivery of chordal implants (Fig. 11) that use sutures and a trans-atrial implantation of a helical anchor, which can then be adjusted to final length postimplantation after weaning from cardiopulmonary bypass.[28] The company was reportedly developing a transcatheter system when it was acquired by Heartware, Inc. In an ovine preclinical model comparing conventional neochords with the device, 8 out of 10 animals in the V-Chordal group had durable resolution of MR at 3 months compared with 2 out of 4 control animals.[20]

SUMMARY

Several transcatheter chordal replacement systems are currently in trial. Many early results are promising; however, data are limited. In order to be successful, a device must demonstrate safety and efficacy compared with surgical repair, with a low burden of chordal/leaflet injury, device failure, device detachment, or residual/recurrent MR.

Decades of surgical data for mitral repair demonstrated that leaflet repair without mitral annuloplasty resulted in an unacceptable burden of recurrent MR owing to annular dilatation over time. Unlike surgical repair, current transcatheter techniques are not designed to prevent ongoing annular dilatation. Transcatheter chordal replacement or leaflet augmentation devices may yet provide options for select patients who are not appropriate for mitral surgery or as a bridge to another therapy. These repair strategies may be able to reduce the burden of MR while still allowing for future transcatheter mitral replacement, which is challenging after TEER. However, these devices are still in development and early preclinical studies, and more data are needed.

CLINICS CARE POINTS

- Transcatheter chordal attachments show promise for minimally-invasive treatment mitral regurgitation.
- Investigational mitral chordal attachments include transcatheter or transapical approaches.
- Multiple clinical trials are ongoing.

DISCLOSURE

Dr G. Lantz serves as an advisor for Edwards Lifesciences and Medtronic, Inc.

REFERENCES

1. Delling FN, Vasan RS. Epidemiology and pathophysiology of mitral valve prolapse: new insights into disease progression, genetics, and molecular basis. Circulation 2014;129:2158–70.
2. Goldstein D, Moskowitz AJ, Gelijns AC, et al. Two-Year Outcomes of Surgical Treatment of Severe Ischemic Mitral Regurgitation. N Engl J Med 2016;374:344–53.
3. Gillinov AM, Blackstone EH, Nowicki ER, et al. Valve repair versus valve replacement for degenerative mitral valve disease. J Thorac Cardiovasc Surg 2008;135:885–93.e2.
4. Hendrix RJ, Bello RA, Flahive JM, et al. Mitral Valve Repair Versus Replacement in Elderly With Degenerative Disease: Analysis of the STS Adult Cardiac Surgery Database. Ann Thorac Surg 2019;107:747–53.
5. Salvador L, Mirone S, Bianchini R, et al. A 20-year experience with mitral valve repair with artificial chordae in 608 patients. J Thorac Cardiovasc Surg 2008;135:1280–7.e1.
6. David TE, Armstrong S, Ivanov J. Chordal replacement with polytetrafluoroethylene sutures for mitral valve repair: A 25-year experience. J Thorac Cardiovasc Surg 2013;145:1563–9.
7. Perier PA. New Paradigm for the Repair of Posterior Leaflet Prolapse: Respect Rather Than Resect. Oper Tech Thorac Cardiovasc Surg 2005;10:180–93.
8. David TE, David CM, Tsang W, et al. Long-Term Results of Mitral Valve Repair for Regurgitation Due to Leaflet Prolapse. J Am Coll Cardiol 2019;74:1044–53.
9. Percutaneous Repair or Surgery for Mitral Regurgitation | NEJM. Available at: https://www.nejm.org/doi/full/10.1056/nejmoa1009355. Accessed July 19, 2023.
10. Stone GW, Lindenfeld J, Abraham WT, et al. Transcatheter Mitral-Valve Repair in Patients with Heart Failure. N Engl J Med 2018;379:2307–18.

11. Zahr F., Mitral Valve Repair With More Natural Physiologic Functionality of the Mitral Valve (Half-Moon). TCTMD.com Available at: https://www.tctmd.com/slide/mitral-valve-repair-more-natural-physiologic-functionality-mitral-valve-half-moon (2021). Accessed September 4, 2023.

12. D'Onofrio A, Fiocco A, Nadali M, et al. Transapical mitral valve repair procedures: Primetime for microinvasive mitral valve surgery. J Card Surg 2022;37:4053–61.

13. Gerosa G, Nadali M, Longinotti L, et al. Transapical off-pump echo-guided mitral valve repair with neochordae implantation mid-term outcomes. Ann Cardiothorac Surg 2021;10:131–40.

14. D'Onofrio A, Mastro F, Nadali M, et al. Transapical beating heart mitral valve repair versus conventional surgery: a propensity-matched study. Interact Cardiovasc Thorac Surg 2022;35:ivac053.

15. NeoChord. Randomized Trial of the NeoChordTM DS1000TM System Versus Open Surgical Repair. Available at: https://clinicaltrials.gov/study/NCT02803957 (2019). Accessed July 12, 2023.

16. Gammie JS, Bartus K, Gackowski A, et al. Beating-Heart Mitral Valve Repair Using a Novel ePTFE Cordal Implantation Device: A Prospective Trial. J Am Coll Cardiol 2018;71:25–36.

17. Gammie JS, Bartus K, Gackowski A, et al. Safety and performance of a novel transventricular beating heart mitral valve repair system: 1-year outcomes. Eur J Cardio Thorac Surg 2021;59:199–206.

18. Wang S, Meng X, Luo Z, et al. Transapical Beating-Heart Mitral Valve Repair Using a Novel Artificial Chordae Implantation System. Ann Thorac Surg 2018;106:e265–7.

19. Wang S, Meng X, Hu S, et al. Initial experiences of transapical beating-heart mitral valve repair with a novel artificial chordal implantation device. J Card Surg 2022;37:1242–9.

20. Maisano F, Cioni M, Seeburger J, et al. Beating-heart implantation of adjustable length mitral valve chordae: acute and chronic experience in an animal model. Eur J Cardiothorac Surg 2011;40:840–7.

21. Bolling S.F., LATE BREAKING FIM – First Case of PIPELINE Chordal Replacement. TCTMD.com. Available at: https://www.tctmd.com/slide/late-breaking-fim-first-case-pipeline-chordal-replacement (2019). Accessed September 11, 2023.

22. Rogers JH, Ebner AA, Boyd WD, et al. First-in-Human Transfemoral Transseptal Mitral Valve Chordal Repair. JACC Cardiovasc Interv 2020;13:1383–5.

23. Rinaldi, M. Transseptal Transcatheter Mitral Valve Chordal Repair Using the CardioMech Valve Repair System: Early First in Human Experience. in TCTMD.com (2021).

24. Weber A, Carrel T, Maisano F, et al. TCT-635 Transcatheter Mitral Repair With a Sutureless Neochordal Device: Preclinical Experience. J Am Coll Cardiol 2016;68:B258.

25. Weber A, Taramasso M, Podkopajev A, et al. Mitral valve repair with a device for artificial chordal implantation at 2 years. JTCVS Open 2021;8:280–9.

26. Latib A, Ho EC, Scotti A, et al. First-in-Human Transseptal Transcatheter Mitral Chordal Repair. JACC Cardiovasc Interv 2022;15:1768–9.

27. Ticar JM, Gaidulis G, Veith K, et al. Mitral Butterfly. JACC Basic Transl Sci 2020;5:1002–14.

28. Fiocco A, Nadali M, Speziali G, et al. Transcatheter Mitral Valve Chordal Repair: Current Indications and Future Perspectives. Front Cardiovasc Med 2019;6.

Transcatheter Therapy for Mitral Valve Stenosis

Kris Kumar, DO, MSc*, Timothy Simpson, PharmD, MD

KEYWORDS

- Transcatheter therapies • Mitral valve stenosis • Rheumatic valvular disease
- Structural cardiology

KEY POINTS

- Mitral valve stenosis remains an important form of valvular heart disease albeit with changing etiology and prevalence in the developed world.
- An in-depth understanding of the anatomic and physiologic effects of rheumatic and non-rheumatic forms is required for delivering optimal transcatheter therapies.
- Percutaneous balloon valvotomy remains a safe and effective therapy for many patients with rheumatic mitral stenosis.
- Ongoing advancements in transcatheter mitral valve replacement may enhance therapeutic options for valvular stenosis in patients with bioprosthetic valve degeneration, annular calcification, or prior mitral annuloplasty.

INTRODUCTION

Mitral valve stenosis remains highly prevalent among the US population although with dramatically shifting demographics. The significance of rheumatic mitral disease in developing nations persists, despite improvements in preventative measures and early detection, and its presence in developed countries is still evident as observed through international migration. In addition, the substantial growth in the aging population with a heightened occurrence of concurrent cardiovascular risk factors is leading to an increased prevalence of chronic calcific degeneration and degeneration of previously repaired or replaced valves.[1] This shift in demographics and causative factors are prompting changes in both diagnosis and treatment methods. In either form, mitral stenosis leads to left atrial enlargement, atrial fibrillation, development of clinical heart failure, and when left untreated is associated with poor outcomes. Initially, medical therapy is used to alleviate symptoms related to mitral stenosis; however, this has not shown significant benefit in altering the long-term outcomes of the disease.[2] Therefore, structural intervention among indicated and eligible patients, a population which remains severely undertreated, affords the best opportunity for improvement of quality of life and longevity.

Pathophysiology of Mitral Stenosis

The differences between rheumatic and non-rheumatic mitral stenosis are vast. In consideration for structural interventions, it is best to consider both as separate entities for which implementing the ideal strategy requires a deeper understanding of mitral valve anatomy and pathology.

The mitral valve is a considerably more complex anatomic structure than its aortic counterpart, consisting of a dynamic saddle-shaped mitral annulus, leaflets, chordae tendinea, and papillary muscles. The mitral valve orifice in its normal state encompasses an area of 4 to 6 cm^2 which effectively establishes a shared cavity between the left atrium and the left ventricle during the diastolic phase of the cardiac cycle. During the early diastole, a transitory, minor

---

Oregon Health and Science University, Portland, OR, USA
* Corresponding author.
E-mail address: kumarkri@ohsu.edu

Intervent Cardiol Clin 13 (2024) 271–278
https://doi.org/10.1016/j.iccl.2024.01.003
2211-7458/24/© 2024 Elsevier Inc. All rights reserved.

pressure gradient emerges between the left atrium and left ventricle, which rapidly equilibrates, rendering both chambers nearly isobaric for the majority of the filling phase.

In the context of mitral stenosis, the constriction of the mitral orifice impedes transit of blood from the left atrium to the left ventricle. This impingement begets the genesis of a discernible pressure gradient between these two cardiac chambers. The superimposed pressure gradient is summated with the intrinsic left ventricular diastolic pressure. Consequently, a heightened left atrial pressure ensues, eventually resulting in left atrial dilatation and the consequent development of pulmonary congestion. As the severity of stenosis intensifies, the constriction of blood flow exerts a restrictive influence on the left ventricular output. The clinical manifestations resemble those associated with left ventricular insufficiency, encompassing pulmonary congestion and a concomitant reduction in cardiac output. Importantly, despite similar sequelae, the mechanism of valvular stenosis is markedly different between rheumatic and non-rheumatic etiologies.

Rheumatic heart disease (RHD) occurs following infection with beta-hemolytic Group A Streptococcus (GAS) and subsequent rheumatic fever which alters the immune response leading to deformities in valve structure and function.[3] RHD is estimated to affect 15 million people worldwide, contributing more than 250,000 new cases yearly and is responsible for more than 200,000 deaths yearly.[4] Most of the cases of RHD occur in endemic regions without readily available access to health care or financial resources to support recognition of symptoms of rheumatic fever or treatment with salicylates and secondary prevention via antibiotics, oftentimes penicillin. Diagnosis of rheumatic fever is classically identified via the Jones criteria, developed by Dr Duckett Jones in 1944, which includes major and minor criteria for diagnosis in addition to recent infection with GAS via laboratory confirmation (Table 1).[5] Carditis, one of the major criteria, initially was identified via physical examination, either via murmur, friction rub, or at later stages decompensated heart failure secondary to valvular heart disease. Pathophysiology of the cardiac manifestations of valvular involvement in RHD is thought to be due to abnormal immunologic response to GAS infection causing an autoimmune inflammatory cascade affecting multiple organ systems.[6,7] It is believed that the M-protein antigen of rheumatic fever is responsible for immune system-mediated response toward valvular structures

Table 1	
Jones criteria for diagnosis of rheumatic fever	
Major Criteria	**Minor Criteria**
Carditis	Polyarthralgia
Polyarthritis	Fever* $\geq$ 38.5°C
Chorea	Elevated inflammatory markers
Erythema marginatum	First-degree aortic valve (AV) block
Subcutaneous nodules	

* Diagnosis via 2 major criteria or 1 major criteria + 2 minor criteria.

of the heart, often aortic and mitral valve disease. The autoimmune cascade then begins the inflammatory process which leads to thickening and scarring of the heart valves and subsequent valvular dysfunction due to commissural fusion.[8]

In contrast, mitral annular calcification as a protypical non-rheumatic etiology is a consequent of chronic and progressive noninfectious inflammation with resulting remodeling and calcification affecting the fibrous mitral annulus and, when severe, the mitral valve leaflets leading to impingement.[9] Risk factors associated with mitral annular calcification (MAC) encompass advanced age, female gender, chronic kidney disease, and conditions predisposing individuals to left ventricular hypertrophy, including hypertension and aortic stenosis.[10] The multifactorial nature of MAC is underscored by a diverse interplay of abnormal calcium and phosphorus metabolism, heightened hemodynamic stress on the mitral valve, and atherosclerotic processes.[11]

Hemodynamic Consequences

In rheumatic MS, chronic immune-mediated inflammation results in leaflet-edge thickening and leads to commissural fusion, with the greatest narrowing at the leaflet tips resulting in a funnel-shaped stenotic orifice. In contrast, mitral annular calcification as a protypical non-rheumatic etiology involves the annulus and base of the leaflets, resulting in a tubular stenotic orifice. Hemodynamically, rheumatic mitral stenosis (MS) leads to increased resistance at the leaflet tips that may be reflected by a blunted left atrial y descent along with persistent diastolic separation of atrioventricular pressures. In contrast, MAC often leads to an elevated left atrial V wave, followed by rapid y descent with equilibration of the atrioventricular pressures, indicating elevated impedance to flow and highlighting the complexity that non-inflow obstruction factors may contribute to such hemodynamics.[12] These subtle, but important differences, may help inform employment of the most optimal transcatheter therapy for such patients.

TREATMENT OF RHEUMATIC MITRAL STENOSIS

Medical therapy for treatment of RHD includes aimed at the symptomatic management of volume overload with diuretics as well as treatment of heart failure via guideline-directed medical therapy as well as rate control to improve diastolic filling time and improve forward flow in rheumatic mitral stenosis.[13] However, the definitive treatment for rheumatic mitral stenosis is either via surgical or transcatheter options. Identification of which therapy to provide patients with RHD is best done at experienced heart valve centers via consultation with a heart team involving cardiologists, imaging specialists, interventionalists, and cardiothoracic surgeons.[14] Surgical options for mitral stenosis involve mitral commissurotomy, repair, or replacement of the valve. In patients who develop symptoms related to mitral stenosis, surgical, or transcatheter therapies provide a survival benefit compared with medical therapy alone.[15] In addition, as pulmonary hypertension develops (mean pulmonary artery pressure >20 mm Hg), surgical risk increases as defined by the Society of Thoracic Surgeons risk scores.[16]

BALLOON MITRAL VALVOTOMY

Balloon mitral valvotomy (BMV) remains the preferred therapy of choice in patients with rheumatic mitral stenosis due to commissural fusion and favorable anatomy for intervention without contraindications to therapy (multivalvular pathology benefitting from surgical intervention, left atrial appendage thrombus assessed via trans-esophageal echocardiogram, moderate to severe mitral regurgitation, intolerance to anticoagulation, pregnancy).[17] First developed in Japan by Inoue and colleagues in a series of six consecutive patients, the technique has been refined over the decades to be an alternative to thoracotomy.[18] Percutaneous BMV compared with surgical closed commissurotomy has been shown to have favorable long-term outcomes in multiple trials and is thus the

favored approach.[19,20] In addition, the procedure can be repeated due to recurrent restenosis over time, providing symptomatic relief due to improved hemodynamics without need for surgery.

Assessment of Balloon Mitral Valvotomy Favorability

Scoring systems to assess the favorability of BMV and procedural success have been developed to guide clinicians in patient selection for this transcatheter approach. Noninvasive assessment of valvular structure and the subvalvular apparatus can be graded according to the Wilkins scoring system, assigning a score of 0 to 4 to degree of valvular mobility, subvalvular thickening, leaflet thickening, and degree of valvular calcification (Table 2).[21] Of the 22 patients studied, a combined score of less than 8 indicated an optimal result following BMV, whereas scores greater than 8 indicated suboptimal results defined as elevated left atrial pressure greater than 10 mm Hg, valve area post-BMV less than 1.0 cm^2, or a less than 25% increase of mitral valve area from baseline. Since the original scoring system developed by Wilkins and colleagues, several other scoring systems have been studied to include the risk of mitral regurgitation post-BMV, assessment of commissural calcium deposition, and further stratification of the subvalvular apparatus.[22–25] However, as the scoring systems are based on imaging to determine valve structure and function, there are limitations to the scores as they rely on adequate imaging and observer interpretation. Thus, before valvular intervention, the role of the heart team in assessment of the patient, symptoms, surgical risk, and assessment of procedural success is paramount in assuring optimal outcomes.

Procedural Steps

Transcatheter BMV involves femoral venous access and subsequent transeptal puncture into the left atrium after which a wire can be advanced across the mitral valve into the left ventricle. Following this, a balloon is advanced over the wire into position within the mitral valve and inflated and deflated to improve leaflet mobility of the fused commissures causing valvular stenosis. Intraprocedural echocardiography via transesophageal or intracardiac echocardiography is used to guide transeptal puncture, balloon sizing and inflation as well as further assessment of leaflet movement, mitral valve pressure gradients, and change of mitral valve area and subsequent regurgitation.

Table 2
Wilkins score for assessment of mitral balloon valvotomy

Grade	Mobility	Subvalvular Thickening	Thickening	Calcification
1	Highly mobile	Minimal below leaflets	Normal (4–5 mm)	Single area
2	Mid and base normal	Thickening of chordal structures up to 1/3 of chordal length	Mid leaflet/marginal	Scattered to leaflet margins
3	Diastolic forward movement	Thickening extending to distal third	Total thickening >5 mm	Brightness to mid leaflets
4	None or minimal forward diastolic movement	Extensive thickening to papillary muscles	Severe thickening >8 mm	Extensive brightness to leaflet tissue

Procedural Risks

Procedural risks include those related to invasive procedures as well as the risk of tamponade due to transeptal puncture which may require emergent surgery. Acute mitral regurgitation due to leaflet damage as a result of balloon inflation or wiring may also require surgical intervention. Despite this, technical success remains high with low complication rates.

Outcomes of Balloon Mitral Valvotomy

Patients undergoing BMV demonstrate excellent short- and long-term results. BMV in the initial series from Inoue and colleagues demonstrated mitral valve area improvement from 1.40 to 2.0 cm^2 with significant reduction in left atrial pressure and mean pressure gradients across the mitral valve in patients with pliable leaflets favorable for intervention.[26] Thirty-day outcomes from 24 centers in the United States as part of the National Heart, Lung, and Blood Institute Balloon Valvuloplasty Registry Participants demonstrated a low 30-day mortality rate of 3% with more than 80% reporting improvement in symptoms.[27] In addition, of the 738 patients included in the registry, overall complication rate was 12% with a 1% procedural mortality rate.[28] Ten-year outcomes showing survival of more than 70% and restenosis-free rates of more than 65% at 10-year follow-up.[29] The absence of post-BMV mitral regurgitation has been independently associated with favorable outcomes following BMV in long-term follow-up.[30]

TRANSCATHER MITRAL VALVE REPLACEMENT FOR RHEUMATIC MITRAL STENOSIS

Transcatheter mitral valve replacement (TMVR) is an emerging therapy for many patients with mitral valve disorders through novel valve technologies currently in investigational trials.[31–36]

The use of TMVR devices has not been studied in the RHD population, and the need for a rigid anchor to maintain bioprosthetic position may be problematic. The calcification that is present in patients with MAC to help anchor the TMVR device is oftentimes not present in younger patients with RHD, though this increases with age.[37] Thus, the current usage of TMVR in rheumatic mitral stenosis is limited to case reports among patients without alternative therapeutic options. The development of TMVR devices that account for stability in the setting of commissural fusion at the level of the leaflets without calcification as opposed to mitral annular anchoring is to be considered in design and may eventually be a viable therapy for such patients.[38]

TMVR procedures require assessment of left ventricular outflow tract (LVOT) obstruction via preprocedural computed tomography imaging via reconstruction of a neo-LVOT. Neo-LVOT of less than 190 mm^2 is associated with a higher risk for obstruction, and thus these patients require further procedural planning via either septal laceration, alcohol septal ablation, or resection before proceeding with TMVR.[39] In the development of specific TMVR valves for RHD, these considerations must be considered as well due to the risk of obstruction from valve replacement.

TREATMENT OF NON-RHEUMATIC MITRAL STENOSIS

Numerous etiologies contribute to non-rheumatic mitral valve stenosis, with mitral annular calcification and dysfunction of surgical bioprosthetic valves being predominant in contemporary clinical scenarios.

Severe mitral stenosis due to annular calcification poses significant anatomic challenges to conventional surgical and percutaneous therapies.

Historically, patients with mitral valve dysfunction due to MAC are at high surgical risk, in-part, due to a high burden of comorbid conditions. Surgical intervention is feasible, albeit challenging, and has been associated a roughly sixfold increase in operative mortality as compared with other forms of mitral valve dysfunction with early post-operative mortality as high as 28%.[40] Although demonstrated to be technically feasible, for reasons previously discussed balloon valvuloplasty is often ineffective at providing significant and durable improvement in hemodynamics or clinical symptoms.[41]

The challenges in the management of mitral stenosis due to surgical bioprosthetic dysfunction are mirrored. Balloon valvuloplasty offers little meaningful benefit and the overall operative, 30-day, and 1-year mortality in some populations are estimated at 3.4%, 22.4%, and 25.9%, respectively.[42] Thus, there remains a significant unmet need in the treatment of such patients.

TRANSCATHER MITRAL VALVE REPLACEMENT FOR NON-RHEUMATIC MITRAL STENOSIS

In contrast to transcatheter aortic valve replacement, where rigid and frequently calcified aortic valve leaflets and annulus provide sufficient interaction to anchor sutureless prostheses, the implantation of sutureless mitral prostheses poses unique challenges. Anatomically these include (1) a dynamic D-shaped annulus with significant variability in diameter throughout the cardiac cycle; (2) marked pressure gradients between the left ventricle and left atrium during systole thus increasing the risk of embolization; and (3) risk of injury to adjacent structures and LVOT obstruction.[43]

Despite such anatomic challenges, surgical bioprostheses, many annuloplasty rings, and certain highly calcified mitral annuli can act as effective anchors for TMVR. The first valve-in-valve (ViV) TMVR in humans took place in 2019 via a transapical approach.[44] This technique was later expanded to address patients with deteriorating rings (valve-in-ring [ViR]) in 2011 and severe MAC (valve in MAC [ViMAC]) in 2013, and additional new approaches such as transseptal delivery were gradually incorporated. However, although the procedure is similar in the three scenarios, the technical challenges, patient risk profiles, and the risk of complications and suboptimal results vary significantly across the groups.

Among the largest data sets, the early TMVR experience included within the Society of Thoracic Surgeons/American College of Cardiology Transcatheter Valve Therapy Registry explores the different clinical outcomes associated with TMVR in three specific scenarios: ViV, ViMAC, and ViR.[45]

While not specific to mitral stenosis, among the 903 patients included for analysis the majority (67.6%) demonstrated significant mitral stenosis with an average mitral valve area of 1.3 cm^2 and mean transmitral gradient of 11 mm Hg, highlighting an overall significant burden of mitral stenosis and/or mixed valvular disease. Groups differed according to mechanism of failure; mitral gradients were highest among subjects with mitral prosthesis or mitral annular calcification, whereas patients with a previous ring displayed increased instances of mitral regurgitation. Subjects were a median age of 75 years with 59.2% female and nearly 90% demonstrated the New York Heart Association III or IV symptoms.

Technical success was more frequent in ViV as compared with ViR or ViMAC (90.9 vs 82.9 vs 74%, P < .001). Procedural complications including LVOT obstruction, need for second

Table 3
Select transcatheter mitral valve replacement outcomes by etiology

Outcome	Valve-in-Valve (n = 680)	Valve-in-Ring (n = 123)	Valve-In-MAC (n = 100)	
Technical Success	617 (90.9%)	102 (82.9%)	74 (74%)	<0.001
In-hospital death	43 (6.3)	11 (9)	18 (18%)	0.004
Mortality, 30 d	47 (8.1%)	12 (11.5%)	20 (20%)	0.003
Device embolization	1 (0.2%)	3 (3.6%)	1 (1.0%)	0.014
LVOT obstruction	5 (0.7%)	6 (4.9%)	10 (10%)	<0.001
Mitral valve reintervention	2 (0.4%)	1 (1.2%)	4 (6.3%)	0.002

From the Society of Thoracic Surgeons/American College of Cardiology Transcatheter Valve Therapy Registry.

valve, all-cause in-hospital mortality, and need for reintervention were generally higher among patients undergoing ViMAC (Table 3). The median postprocedure mitral valve gradient among the cohort was 4 mm Hg and most had mild residual mitral regurgitation (MR) or less. The overall all-cause mortality during the study period was 10.1%.

This early registry experience suggests TMVR to be a technically feasible therapy among patients with a reasonable incidence of procedural complication. Of note, there were significant differences in the rates of procedural success and periprocedural complications among different forms of mitral valve disease, highlighting the need for an in-depth understanding of the anatomic and physiologic characterization of such patients to maintain high-efficiency outcomes. Further dispersion of transseptal delivery and dedicated TMVR devices may further drive procedural success and safety.

SUMMARY

Mitral valve stenosis remains an important form of valvular heart disease albeit with changing etiology and prevalence among an aging population in the developed world. The complex features of mitral valve stenosis and the distinct anatomic and pathophysiologic manifestations of rheumatic and non-rheumatic etiologies pose a challenge to clinicians. Devising the optimal strategy for percutaneous intervention among such patients requires in-depth understanding and tailored approach on the bases of such principals. The growing availability of TMVR poses a unique opportunity, when properly applied, for improved outcomes in such patients.

CLINICS CARE POINTS

- Identification of valvular heart disease is crucial to improve patient outcomes.

- Mitral stenosis can lead to acute and chronic decompensated heart failure when left untreated can lead to poor patient outcomes.

- Among eligible patients, transcatheter therapies such as balloon mitral valvotomy remains the perfered therapy of choice for rheumatic mitral stenosis.

- Investigation of other transcatheter therapies is ongoing to provide further treatment and therapeutic options in this challenging subset of valvular heart disease patients.

DISCLOSURE

All authors report no conflicts of interest, disclosures, or funding sources related to this article. All authors take responsibility for all aspects of the reliability and freedom from bias of the data presented and their discussed interpretation. This research did not receive any specific grant from funding agencies in the public, commercial, or not-for-profit sectors.

REFERENCES

1. Eleid M, Foley TA, Said SM, et al. Severe mitral annular calcification: Multimodality imaging for therapeutic strategies and interventions. JACC Cardiovascular Imaging 2016;9(11):1318–2337.
2. Chandrashekhar Y, Westaby S, Narula J. Mitral stenosis. Lancet 2009;374(9697):1271–83.
3. Dass C, Kanmanthareddy A. In: Rheumatic Heart Disease. In: StatPearls [Internet]. Treasure Island, FL: StatPearls Publishing; 2024.
4. Seckeler MD, Hoke TR. The worldwide epidemiology of acute rheumatic fever and rheumatic heart disease. Clin Epidemiol 2011;3:67–84.
5. JONES TD. The diagnosis of rheumatic fever. J Am Med Assoc 1944;126(8):481–4.
6. Liu M, Lu L, Sun R, et al. Rheumatic Heart Disease: Causes, Symptoms, and Treatments. Cell Biochem Biophys 2015;72(3):861–3.
7. Guilherme L, Kalil J. Rheumatic fever and rheumatic heart disease: cellular mechanisms leading autoimmune reactivity and disease. J Clin Immunol 2010; 30(1):17–23.
8. Kaplan EL. Pathogenesis of acute rheumatic fever and rheumatic heart disease: evasive after half a century of clinical, epidemiological, and laboratory investigation. Heart 2005;91(1):3–4.
9. Korn D, Desanctis R, Sell S. Massive calcification of the mitral annulus- a clinicopathological study of fourteen cases. N Engl J Med 1962;267:900–9.
10. Lee H, Seo J, Gwak S, et al. Risk factors and outcomes with progressive mitral annular calcification. JAHA 2023;12:e030620.
11. Eleid M, Foley T, Said S, et al. Severe mitral annular calcification: multimodality imaging for therapeutic strategies and interventions. JACC Cardiovasc Imaging 2016;9(11):1318–37.
12. Reddy Y, Murgo J, Nishimura R. Complexity of defining severe stenosis from mitral annular calcification. Circulation 2019;149(7):523–5.
13. Kumar RK, Antunes MJ, Beaton A, et al. Contemporary Diagnosis and Management of Rheumatic Heart Disease: Implications for Closing the Gap: A Scientific Statement From the American Heart Association. Circulation 2020;142(20):e337–57.
14. Otto CM, Nishimura RA, Bonow RO, et al. 2020 ACC/AHA Guideline for the Management of

Patients With Valvular Heart Disease: A Report of the American College of Cardiology/American Heart Association Joint Committee on Clinical Practice Guidelines. Circulation 2021;143(5):e72–227.

15. Roy SB, Gopinath N. Mitral stenosis. Circulation 1968;38(1 Suppl):68–76.

16. Vincens JJ, Temizer D, Post JR, et al. Long-term outcome of cardiac surgery in patients with mitral stenosis and severe pulmonary hypertension. Circulation 1995;92(9 Suppl):Ii137–42.

17. Carabello BA. Modern management of mitral stenosis. Circulation 2005;112(3):432–7.

18. Inoue K, Owaki T, Nakamura T, et al. Clinical application of transvenous mitral commissurotomy by a new balloon catheter. J Thorac Cardiovasc Surg 1984;87(3):394–402.

19. Ben Farhat M, Ayari M, Maatouk F, et al. Percutaneous balloon versus surgical closed and open mitral commissurotomy: seven-year follow-up results of a randomized trial. Circulation 1998;97(3):245–50.

20. Reyes VP, Raju BS, Wynne J, et al. Percutaneous balloon valvuloplasty compared with open surgical commissurotomy for mitral stenosis. N Engl J Med 1994;331(15):961–7.

21. Wilkins GT, Weyman AE, Abascal VM, et al. Percutaneous balloon dilatation of the mitral valve: an analysis of echocardiographic variables related to outcome and the mechanism of dilatation. Br Heart J 1988;60(4):299–308.

22. Bhalgat P, Karlekar S, Modani S, et al. Subvalvular apparatus and adverse outcome of balloon valvotomy in rheumatic mitral stenosis. Indian Heart J 2015;67(5):428–33.

23. Cannan CR, Nishimura RA, Reeder GS, et al. Echocardiographic assessment of commissural calcium: a simple predictor of outcome after percutaneous mitral balloon valvotomy. J Am Coll Cardiol 1997;29(1):175–80.

24. Nunes MC, Tan TC, Elmariah S, et al. The echo score revisited: Impact of incorporating commissural morphology and leaflet displacement to the prediction of outcome for patients undergoing percutaneous mitral valvuloplasty. Circulation 2014;129(8):886–95.

25. Padial LR, Abascal VM, Moreno PR, et al. Echocardiography can predict the development of severe mitral regurgitation after percutaneous mitral valvuloplasty by the Inoue technique. Am J Cardiol 1999;83(8):1210–3.

26. Nobuyoshi M, Hamasaki N, Kimura T, et al. Indications, complications, and short-term clinical outcome of percutaneous transvenous mitral commissurotomy. Circulation 1989;80(4):782–92.

27. Multicenter experience with balloon mitral commissurotomy. NHLBI Balloon Valvuloplasty Registry Report on immediate and 30-day follow-up results. The National Heart, Lung, and Blood Institute Balloon Valvuloplasty Registry Participants. Circulation 1992;85(2):448–61.

28. Complications and mortality of percutaneous balloon mitral commissurotomy. A report from the National Heart, Lung, and Blood Institute Balloon Valvuloplasty Registry. Circulation 1992;85(6):2014–24.

29. Ben-Farhat M, Betbout F, Gamra H, et al. Predictors of long-term event-free survival and of freedom from restenosis after percutaneous balloon mitral commissurotomy. Am Heart J 2001;142(6):1072–9.

30. Kang DH, Park SW, Song JK, et al. Long-term clinical and echocardiographic outcome of percutaneous mitral valvuloplasty: randomized comparison of Inoue and double-balloon techniques. J Am Coll Cardiol 2000;35(1):169–75.

31. Alperi A, Dagenais F, Del Val D, et al. Early Experience With a Novel Transfemoral Mitral Valve Implantation System in Complex Degenerative Mitral Regurgitation. JACC Cardiovasc Interv 2020;13(20):2427–37.

32. Webb JG, Murdoch DJ, Boone RH, et al. Percutaneous Transcatheter Mitral Valve Replacement: First-in-Human Experience With a New Transseptal System. J Am Coll Cardiol 2019;73(11):1239–46.

33. Zahr F, Song HK, Chadderdon S, et al. 1-Year Outcomes Following Transfemoral Transseptal Transcatheter Mitral Valve Replacement: Intrepid TMVR Early Feasibility Study Results. JACC Cardiovasc Interv 2023;16(23):2868–79.

34. Zahr F, Song HK, Chadderdon SM, et al. 30-Day Outcomes Following Transfemoral Transseptal Transcatheter Mitral Valve Replacement: Intrepid TMVR Early Feasibility Study Results. JACC Cardiovasc Interv 2022;15(1):80–9.

35. Nunes Ferreira-Neto A, Dagenais F, Bernier M, et al. Transcatheter Mitral Valve Replacement With a New Supra-Annular Valve: First-in-Human Experience With the AltaValve System. JACC Cardiovasc Interv 2019;12(2):208–9.

36. Alperi A, Granada JF, Bernier M, et al. Current Status and Future Prospects of Transcatheter Mitral Valve Replacement: JACC State-of-the-Art Review. J Am Coll Cardiol 2021;77(24):3058–78.

37. Guerrero M, Urena M, Himbert D, et al. 1-Year Outcomes of Transcatheter Mitral Valve Replacement in Patients With Severe Mitral Annular Calcification. J Am Coll Cardiol 2018;71(17):1841–53.

38. Weich H, Herbst P, Smit F, et al. Transcatheter heart valve interventions for patients with rheumatic heart disease. Front Cardiovasc Med 2023;10:1234165.

39. Wang DD, Eng MH, Greenbaum AB, et al. Validating a prediction modeling tool for left ventricular

outflow tract (LVOT) obstruction after transcatheter mitral valve replacement (TMVR). Cathet Cardiovasc Interv 2018;92(2):379–87.

40. Alexis S, Malik A, El-Eshmawi A, et al. Surgical and transcatheter mitral valve replacement in mitral annular calcification: A systematic review. JAHA 2021;10(7):e018514.

41. Donatelle M, Patel R, Adasthi P, et al. Off-label use of balloon mitral valvuloplasty in nonrheumatic mitral stenosis with severe mitral annular calcification. JSCAI 2022;1(2):100026.

42. Zubarevich A, Szczechowicz M, Zhigalov K, et al. Surgical redo mitral valve replacement in high-risk patients: The real-world experience. J Card Surg 2021;36(9):3195–204.

43. Urena M, Vahanian A, Brochet E, et al. Current indications for transcatheter mitral valve replacement using transcatheter aortic valves. Circulation 2021;143:178–96.

44. Cheung A, Webb J, Wong D, et al. Transapical transcatheter mitral valve-in-valve implantation in a human. Ann Thorac Surg 2009;87(3):18–20.

45. Guerrero M, Vemulapalli S, Xiang Q, et al. Thirty-day outcomes of transcatheter mitral valve replacement for degenerated mitral vioprosthesis (valve-in-valve), failed surgical rings (valve-in-ring), and native valve with severe mitral annular calcification (valve-in-mitral annular calcification) in the united states. Circ Interventions 2020;13:e008425.

Transcatheter Treatment of Mitral Valve Regurgitation in the Setting of Concomitant Coronary or Multivalvular Heart Disease: A Focused Review

Jay Ramsay, MD[a], Yicheng Tang, MD[b],
Jin Kyung Kim, MD, PhD[b],
Antonio H. Frangieh, MD, MPH[b],*

KEYWORDS

- Mixed valvular heart disease • Percutaneous intervention • Tricuspid regurgitation
- Mitral regurgitation • Aortic stenosis • Aortic regurgitation • Transcatheter edge-to-edge repair

KEY POINTS

- This article summarizes the current literature and guidelines on transcatheter treatment of mitral valve regurgitation in the setting of other coronary or multivalvular heart disease in inoperable patients.
- All patients should be evaluated by a heart team on a case-by-case basis.
- When percutaneous intervention is indicated, a staged approach with serial reevaluation is generally favorable to a single-session approach.
- The order of which valve to intervene on first should take into account the hemodynamic interactions of each valvulopathy.

INTRODUCTION

The function and anatomy of the mitral valve apparatus are complex. The mitral valve is responsible for passively allowing left ventricular (LV) filling during diastole and, more impressively, preventing regurgitation under the high LV pressures of systole.[1] The valve competency owes to the intricate, harmonious coordination of the mitral annulus, leaflets, chordae, and papillary muscles of the mitral apparatus and ideal left atrium and ventricle anatomy and function. When the valve becomes dysfunctional, clinical consequences are serious. In particular, those with mitral valve disease with other valvular pathologies or concomitant coronary artery disease are at high risk of developing heart failure and have high mortality rates.[2–6] Treatment of mixed valve disease has historically been limited, often surgery being the only option. Fortunately, with the recent advancement of transcatheter technology, less invasive percutaneous approaches are quickly becoming viable therapeutic considerations. However, with the emergence of many novel technologies targeting the aortic, mitral, and tricuspid valves, finding the ideal permutation of treatment strategy for those with mixed valvular disease is

[a] Department of Internal Medicine, University of California Irvine, 333 City Boulevard West, City Tower Suite 400, Orange, CA 92868, USA; [b] Division of Cardiology, University of California Irvine, 333 City Boulevard West, City Tower Suite 400, Orange, CA 92868, USA
* Corresponding author. Division of Cardiology, Departmen of Medicine, University of California Irvine, 333 City Boulevard West, City Tower Suite 400, Orange, CA 92868.
E-mail address: afrangie@hs.uci.edu

Intervent Cardiol Clin 13 (2024) 279–289
https://doi.org/10.1016/j.iccl.2023.12.005

daunting. Guidelines on managing this particularly complex set of patients are sparse because of insufficient data, discrepancies among available data, and significant patient heterogeneity. In addition, multiple interventions of mixed valvular disease in a single session may introduce logistical hurdles in the catheterization laboratories and health care systems without established long-term benefits.

This review summarizes the current literature on percutaneous interventions (PCI) of mitral regurgitation (MR) in the setting of mixed valvular or coronary artery disease, with a focus on pathophysiology, and the timing and order of interventions.

AORTIC STENOSIS AND MITRAL REGURGITATION

Up to 20% of patients with severe aortic stenosis (AS) have concomitant severe MR.[5,7] Patients with moderate-to-severe MR and severe AS have higher mortality than those with severe AS alone.[8] Evaluation of patients with mixed AS and MR is made difficult by the hemodynamic relationship between the two valvular lesions. AS causes increased LV afterload, leading to LV hypertrophy and concentric remodeling. As the disease advances, the LV and mitral annulus dilate causing secondary MR (Fig. 1). However, the regurgitant volume of MR decreases forward flow through the left ventricle, lowering the forward stroke volume, which can underestimate the severity of AS by relatively lowering aortic valve gradient.[9,10] Historically, patients undergoing cardiac surgery for concomitant MR and AS face a 15.5% in-hospital mortality rate and median lifespan of 7.3 years.[11] The advent of transcatheter aortic valve replacement (TAVR) and percutaneous mitral valve therapies, such as mitral transcatheter edge-to-edge repair (M-TEER), opened the possibility of intervention to many who pose a prohibitive surgical risk and otherwise had no options and with unprecedented results. Unlike surgery where intervention on the aortic and mitral valve should clearly be done in the same session, these transcatheter approaches introduce the option to intervene in series.[12,13]

Although the optimal order of procedures needs to be individualized, and the ideal wait time between procedures is still unclear, the sequence of interventions should prioritize the downstream aortic valve. If the MR is treated first, the AS-induced LV afterload might cause LV failure. Both the 2020 American College of Cardiology/American Heart Association (ACC/AHA) and 2021 European Society of Cardiology/European Association for Cardiothoracic Surgery (ESC/EACTS) guidelines recommend that prohibitive-risk patients with severe AS and severe MR should undergo staged TAVR first followed by M-TEER if symptomatic MR persists.[12,13] Of note, the guidelines do not differ on primary versus secondary MR. Although MR improves approximately half of the time after TAVR,[5,8,14] data show that secondary MR is more likely to improve after TAVR than primary MR.[14,15] Factors associated with a lower likelihood of MR improvement include atrial fibrillation, mitral annular calcification, left atrial diameter greater than 5 cm, LV end-systolic diameter less than 45 mm, and preoperative peak aortic valve gradient less than 60 mm Hg.[16–20] Witberg and colleagues[14] also showed in the retrospective Aortic + Mitral TRAnsCatheter (AMTRAC) Registry that patients whose MR persisted after TAVR carried significantly higher 4-year mortality than those whose MR improved after TAVR (43.8% vs 35.1%). Of those whose MR persisted, staged M-TEER post-TAVR was associated with a better 1-year New York Heart Association (NYHA) functional class (82.4% vs 33.3% NYHA I/II) and trended toward lower 4-year mortality (64.6% vs 37.5%; hazard ratio, 1.66; $P = .097$).[14] Interpretation of these data is limited by different grading methods used to assess MR severity, lack of centralized and adjudicated echocardiography data, and variable follow-up periods among the studies.

There are no clear data on the optimal time to proceed with M-TEER after TAVR, and the decision should ultimately be based on each patient's specific clinical needs. A retrospective analysis of 626 patients undergoing M-TEER and TAVR compared outcomes of those who had the procedures done during separate verse the same admission.[21] After adjusting for age, sex, and comorbidities, they found that although the overall mortality rates between the two groups were similar, those who had both procedures during the same admission had higher rates of acute kidney injury, vascular complications, need for PCI, mechanical support, and pacemaker insertion. Although the study did not quantify the number of days between procedures, it is safely assumed patients who had both interventions during the same admission had fewer days between interventions than those who were treated in two separate hospitalizations. The AMTRAC registry reported a median of 61 days from TAVR to M-TEER.[14] Even less data exist on single-session TAVR and M-TEER. Rudolph and colleagues[22]

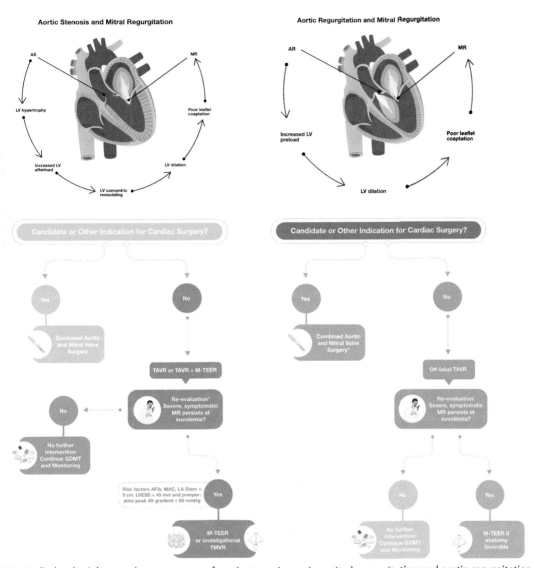

Fig. 1. Pathophysiology and management of aortic stenosis causing mitral regurgitation and aortic regurgitation causing mitral regurgitation. * Surgery for severe aortic regurgitation when it is symptomatic (1B-NR), causing LV systolic dysfunction (1B-NR), already undergoing cardiac surgery (1C-EO), or when LV is severely enlarged (2a B-NR). A Fib, atrial fibrillation; AV, aortic valve; LA, left atrium; LVESD, left ventricle end-systolic dimension; MAC, mitral annular calcification.

reported their experience with three patients, showing that a single-session TAVR and M-TEER is feasible. In all three cases, TAVR preceded the M-TEER. They also reported one case of M-TEER 10 days before TAVR. Witberg and colleagues[23] reported 100% technical success of concomitant TAVR and transcatheter mitral intervention (2 M-TEER, 3 mitral valve-in-valve, and 1 transcatheter heart valve in the mitral position) from the German transcatheter mitral valve interventions (TRAMI) registry. The outcomes of the six patients who had TAVR and transcatheter mitral valve replacement/

repair (TMVR/r) were comparable with those who underwent staged intervention from the same registry, although data are susceptible to small sample bias.[23] More research is needed to further assess the benefits and risks of single-session TAVR and TMVR/r.

In summary, evidence supports that symptomatic patients with severe AS and greater than or equal to 2+ MR who are deemed appropriate for transcatheter intervention first undergo TAVR with close reevaluation of the MR post-TAVR, then proceed with staged M-TEER if significant MR persists (see **Fig. 1**). Optimal timing between the two interventions is yet to be established. Given scant data, it is yet difficult to draw a firm conclusion on the benefits of concomitant TAVR and M-TEER in a single session.

AORTIC REGURGITATION AND MITRAL REGURGITATION

The prevalence of combined aortic regurgitation (AR) and MR varies wildly across populations.[24,25] Up to a quarter of patients with severe AR also have moderate-to-severe MR.[26,27] The increased preload in chronic AR can result in LV remodeling and dilation (see Fig. 1). This then impacts the mitral apparatus, leading to poor coaptation of the mitral leaflets and secondary MR.[28] When the aortic valve is replaced surgically, the secondary MR improves by at least one grade in most (~90%) patients.[29] Guidelines currently recommend surgical intervention for severe AR causing symptoms, LV systolic dysfunction, during concomitant cardiac surgery, or when LV is severely enlarged.[12] For patients who are not candidates for surgery, TAVR is an off-label option with results comparable with surgical aortic valve replacement.[30,31] TAVR for AR is technically challenging, and size selection must weigh the risks of dislocation and oversizing. A predominantly regurgitant aortic valve may lack significant calcification the standard TAVR valves depend on for stable anchoring.[12,30] Recently, novel technologies, such as the percutaneous leaflet-capturing Trilogy system that does not require calcification for anchoring, received a CE (European Conformity) mark for the treatment of AR.[32] Prospective data of the Trilogy system will soon be available from the Align AR trial.[33]

Current data on PCI for severe AR and severe MR are limited to case reports in the last 10 years. Most often, it is treated in stages with the TAVR done before M-TEER. Only one case report of a successful single-session TAVR and valve-in-valve TMVR has been reported.[34] A successful single-session TAVR and chord repair for severe AR and MR with mitral annular calcification has also been reported using the Neochord DS 100 device.[35] In another case, a successful single-session TAVR, followed by intra-aortic balloon pump, then M-TEER was reported for a patient with cardiogenic shock from a late-presenting ST segment elevated myocardial infarction with severe AR and MR.[36] In all three of these cases of single-session intervention, the aortic valve was intervened before the mitral valve. Intervening on the downstream aortic valve may decrease LV preload and create

a more favorable pressure gradient across the mitral valve.[28] Additionally, the LV reverse remodeling may improve the ventricular geometry and mitral subvalvular apparatus, allowing for better mitral valve coaptation and reduction of MR.[29] To our knowledge, there has only been one case report of M-TEER done before off-label TAVR for AR.[37] The patient had multiple comorbidities including chronic arterial dissection from the carotid arteries to the bilateral femoral arteries. The authors stated that they chose to do M-TEER before TAVR because MR was more severe than the AR initially and the technical difficulties related to the arterial access needed for TAVR in the setting of extensive dissection. AR became more severe on a follow-up echocardiography and a successful TAVR was done in a transapical approach.

In summary, cardiac surgery is still the current standard of care for concomitant severe AR and MR, with TAVR considered as an off-label option for those with favorable anatomy who are not candidates for surgery (see Fig. 1). However, the transcatheter technology is rapidly evolving, and novel devices and valve systems designed specifically for nonsurgical treatment of AR are being tested. Completion of these trials, data publication and analysis, and further research will advance the transcatheter-based treatment of mixed valve disease of MR and AR.

TRICUSPID REGURGITATION AND MITRAL REGURGITATION

Moderate or severe tricuspid regurgitation (TR) has a prevalence of up to 30% in those with severe secondary MR.[2] The presence of secondary TR independently confers a worse prognosis.[38,39] Many severe TR cases are secondary to left-sided heart disease including aortomitral valvular dysfunction, LV cardiomyopathy, and/or pulmonary hypertension.[40] Significant secondary TR develops via several mechanisms, with tricuspid annular dilatation often as the common final pathway. Secondary TR is categorized into either atrial-predominant phenotype, which is typically driven by chronic atrial fibrillation with right atrial dilatation, or ventricular-predominant phenotype, which is caused by pulmonary hypertension or secondary to left-sided valvular or ventricular disease.[41–43] The timing and approach to intervention for both phenotypes remains unclear, especially as it pertains to novel percutaneous therapies. Primary TR etiology is less frequent. It includes degenerative disease, healed endocarditis, traumatic leaflet tear or perforation, and pacemaker lead impingement. This entity is less likely to change after mitral valve treatment. This section discusses proposed stratification for cases of concomitant secondary TR and MR.

Surgical tricuspid valve repair has existed since Carpentier and colleagues[44] described safety and efficacy of tricuspid ring annuloplasty in 1974. The most recent ESC/EACTS 2021 and ACC/AHA 2020 guidelines recommend that those who are already undergoing left-sided valve surgery should have concomitant surgical intervention for severe secondary TR (class 1) or mild or moderate TR with an annulus greater than 40 mm (class 2a) (Fig. 2).[12,13]

For inoperable patients, there has been a recent expansion of transcatheter options for TR. These include leaflet approximation, annuloplasty, orthotopic valve implantation, and heterotopic valve implantation.[45] Although not mentioned in the 2020 ACC/AHA guidelines, it is a class 2b recommendation by the ESC/EACTS to undergo transcatheter tricuspid valve intervention (TTVI) for severe, symptomatic secondary TR in inoperable patients.[13] This was largely based on the 2019 retrospective analysis of 472 patients in the TriValve registry showing patients who underwent TTVI had lower 1-year all-cause mortality (23% vs 36%) and fewer rehospitalizations for heart failure (26% vs 47%).[46] Subsequently, a 2022 meta-analysis of 1216 patients undergoing TTVI showed that those who had a reduction in the TR grade to 2+ or less had a 58% risk reduction in 1-year mortality.[47] Prospective data from tricuspid TEER (Triluminate Pivotal study,[48] CLASP TR trial[49]), tricuspid replacement (TriSCEND trial[50,51]), and TRI-REPAIR study[52] showed that TTVI is safe, improves quality of life, and improves TR severity in 72% to 98% of patients. However, these prospective randomized studies did not show a significant reduction in mortality or heart failure hospitalizations observed in non-randomized studies, at least up to 1-year follow-up. Additionally, it is important to mention that patients with concomitant severe MR were excluded in the Triluminate, CLASP TR, and TRISCEND Pivotal studies.[48–50] Further prospective data are needed to shed light on the efficacy of TTVI, particularly as it pertains to patients with multivalvular lesions.

TR often exists as a consequence of MR and improves in 23% to 50% of patients after M-TEER.[53–57] One scenario is that as MR is reduced, left atrial dynamics improve, pulmonary pressures normalize, and ultimately positive right ventricular (RV) remodeling leads to a reduction in tricuspid annulus size and approximation of leaflet coaptation.[58] Risk factors for

lack of TR improvement after M-TEER include the presence of atrial fibrillation, chronic RV dysfunction, large tricuspid annulus size, or significant residual MR after M-TEER (see Fig. 2).[59]

There are limited data on the timing and sequencing of TTVI and M-TEER. To date, no prospective studies exist comparing single-session M-TEER plus TTVI versus a staged approach. A retrospective analysis of the Tri-Valve and TRAMI registries showed a higher 1-year survival rate (83.6%) with combined TEER compared with isolated M-TEER (66%).[60] This survival benefit of combined tricuspid and M-TEER should be interpreted with caution, given confounding factors inherent to retrospective analysis. For example, the combined TEER group had significantly worse ejection fraction and lower baseline glomerular filtration rate (GFR). Another retrospective analysis of the Tri-Valve registry found that heart failure exacerbations were similar in those who got TTVI combined with M-TEER, compared with TTVI alone.[46] The conflicting data of these retrospective analyses highlights the need for future prospective randomized controlled studies in this patient population.

In addition to the previously mentioned registry data, studies have been performed to understand the safety and efficacy of specific hemodynamic subtypes within the MR TR population. Stocker and colleagues[61] identified increased mortality following TTVI (T-TEER) for patients with combined precapillary and postcapillary pulmonary hypertension (CpPH) compared with those without pulmonary hypertension or isolated postcapillary pulmonary hypertension (IpcPH). In another interrogation of the TriValve registry by Brener and colleagues,[62] noninvasive estimation of RV–pulmonary artery uncoupling by tricuspid annular plane systolic excursion/pulmonary artery systolic pressure less than a median value of 0.406 was associated with increased risk of all-cause mortality at 1 year after TTVI. These two studies support cautious employment or avoidance of TTVI for patients with advanced pulmonary hypertension with resultant RV failure.

In summary, it is advisable to stratify patients by hemodynamic and anatomic profiling during preprocedural planning for PCI of concomitant MR and TR. Right heart catheterization is underused and crucial for the characterization of CpcPH verse IpcPH in this population. Patients presenting with CpcPH and chronic RV systolic failure represent an advanced disease state that may be less tolerant of valvular intervention and are also less likely to reap long-term benefits because of futility. Similar to surgical patients,

Mitral Regurgitation causing Secondary Tricuspid Regurgitation

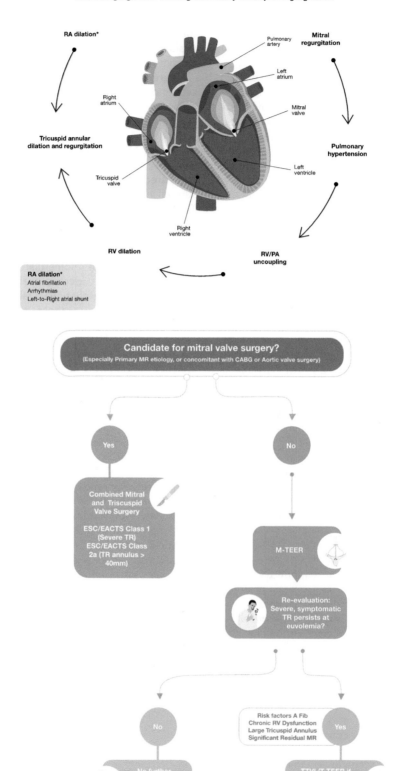

Fig. 2. Pathophysiology and management of mitral regurgitation causing secondary tricuspid regurgitation. * Atrial fibrillation, arrhythmias, and left-to-right atrial shunt. (blue box text). A Fib, atrial fibrillation; CABG, coronary artery bypass graft; PA, pulmonary artery; RA, right atrium; RV, right ventricle; T-TEER, tricuspid transcatheter edge-to-edge repair.

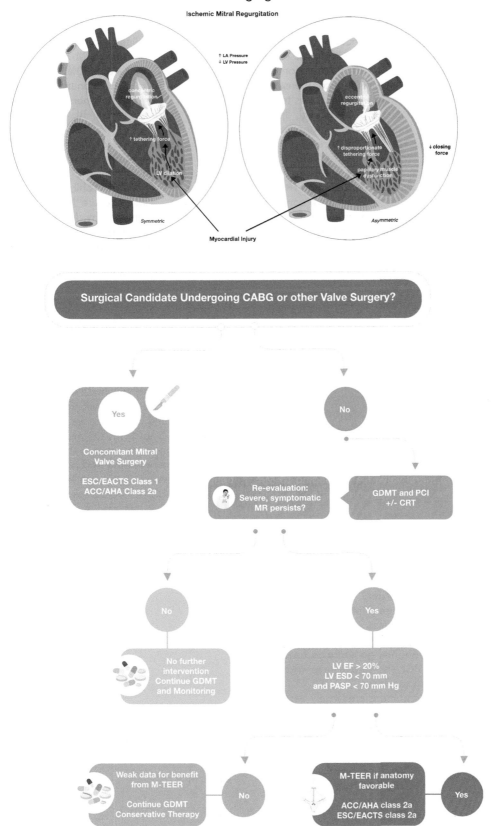

Fig. 3. Pathophysiology and management of ischemic cardiomyopathy causing mitral regurgitation. CABG, coronary artery bypass graft; CRT, cardiac resynchronization therapy; LA, left atrium; LV EF, left ventricular ejection fraction; LV ESD, left ventricle end-systolic dimension; PASP, pulmonary artery systolic pressure.

patients with tenuous RV function may benefit from periprocedural ventricular inotropic drugs, such as milrinone to optimize RV function and reduce the risk of acute RV decompensation that can occur when severe TR improves to less than mild.[63] In contrast, patients with IpcPH may reasonably undergo either concomitant TEER or a staged approach with reassessment of TR following M-TEER. Those with atrial-predominant TR secondary to atrial fibrillation are less likely to achieve a reduction of TR after M-TEER and may gain benefit from a concomitant approach, depending on minimizing procedural time and optimizing resource use. More data on timing, order of interventions, and patient selection regarding transcatheter management of concomitant MR and TR are needed.

ISCHEMIC (CORONARY ARTERY DISEASE) MITRAL REGURGITATION

Ischemic MR starts with coronary artery disease causing pathologic remodeling and dilation of the LV and compromised perfusion to the mitral subvalvular apparatus. The LV dilation is either symmetric or asymmetric. In the former, the mitral annular ring becomes dilated and leads to poor leaflet coaptation. In contrast, the displaced papillary muscles of the asymmetrically dilated LV cause a tethering force on the chordae tendinea mitral valve leaflet leading to MR (Fig. 3). The resulting regurgitation is self-perpetuating because the volume overload from the MR can further exacerbate LV dilation.[64–68] It is an ESC/EACTS class 1 and ACC/AHA class 2a recommendation to have mitral valve surgery for the coexisting severe MR if a patient is undergoing coronary artery bypass graft or other valve surgery.[12,13] For those not eligible for cardiac surgery, M-TEER is an ACC/AHA and ESC/EACTS class 2a recommendation for patients with severe, symptomatic ischemic MR refractory to optimal goal-directed medical therapy (GDMT), PCI, and cardiac resynchronization therapy if indicated (see Fig. 3).[12,13]

These recommendations are largely based on the evidence from the COAPT and MITRA-FR trials.[39,69] In these trials, MitraClip plus GDMT was prospectively compared with GDMT alone for patients with symptomatic MR refractory to optimal GDMT. The COAPT study showed an improvement in survival, hospitalization, symptoms, and quality of life up to 5 years.[70] In contrast to the COAPT trial, the MITRA-FR trial did not show a reduction in the composite end point of death or hospitalization. Because of these differences, and taking into consideration multiple subgroups

analysis, the guidelines adopted these additional criteria for the indication for M-TEER (LV ejection fraction between 20% and 50%, LV end-systolic dimension ≤70 mm, pulmonary artery systolic pressure ≤70 mm Hg, and persistent symptoms [NYHA functional class II, III, or IV] while on optimal GDMT).[12]

The benefits of cardiac surgery for mitral valve replacement or repair for ischemic MR are controversial and outside the scope of this review paper. For high or prohibitive surgical risk patients with primary severe MR in the setting of ischemic cardiomyopathy, M-TEER is reasonable and should not be delayed because the MR is not expected to improve significantly after PCI. Patients should have a life expectancy greater than 1 year and favorable anatomy.[12,13] Ideally, the most favorable anatomy for M-TEER includes a central pathology of the mitral valve, no leaflet calcifications, mitral valve area greater than 4.0 cm2, posterior leaflet greater than 10 mm, tenting height less than 10 mm, flail gap less than 10 mm, and flail width less than 15 mm.[71] With increasing anatomic challenges, M-TEER, although still feasible, requires more operator skill set, and MR reduction is less optimal in some cases. The farther patients are from this ideal anatomy, the more consideration should be given to mitral valve replacement, which is a fast-growing technology.[72] For patients with severe secondary ischemic MR and high or prohibitive surgical risk, the main points of the guidelines are discussed previously. The underlying cause ischemia and the focus should be first on optimizing revascularization, GDMT, and cardiac resynchronization therapy if indicated. If MR remains severe and symptomatic, then M-TEER is indicated with proven mortality and morbidity benefit.

SUMMARY

Patients with MR with other valvular pathologies or concomitant coronary artery disease are clinically complex. Transcatheter therapies targeting the aortic, mitral, and tricuspid valves introduce the option of permutations on order and timing of treatments, with insufficient data to date to recommend single-stage interventions. In general, the order of treatment should prioritize the downstream valve; aortic before mitral and mitral before tricuspid. Ultimately, each patient should be evaluated by a heart team and management should be individualized based on their unique hemodynamics. Further data from large registries and perhaps randomized controlled trials are needed to establish strong evidence-based guidelines.

CLINICS CARE POINTS

- There has been a recent expansion of percutaneous interventions for valvular heart disease. The heart team decision is important in order to consider all options available for their patients, as well as order and timing of interventions.

- In general, the order of percutaneous treatment should prioritize the downstream valve; aortic before mitral and mitral before tricuspid.

- Until there is more data on the safety and efficacy of single-session multivalvular percutaneous interventions, patients should have their valves intervened in sequence with re-evaluation of valve disease severity and symptoms between each procedure.

DISCLOSURE

None of the authors have disclosures.

REFERENCES

1. McCarthy KP, Ring L, Rana BS. Anatomy of the mitral valve: understanding the mitral valve complex in mitral regurgitation. Eur J Echocardiogr 2010;11(10):i3–9.
2. Truong VT, Tam N, Ngo M, et al. Right ventricular dysfunction and tricuspid regurgitation in functional mitral regurgitation. Esc Heart Failure 2021; 8(6):4988–96.
3. Nader M, Diodato MD, Moon MR, et al. Does functional mitral regurgitation improve with isolated aortic valve replacement? J Card Surg 2004;19(5): 444–8.
4. Chakravarty T, Van Belle E, Jilaihawi H, et al. Meta-analysis of the impact of mitral regurgitation on outcomes after transcatheter aortic valve implantation. Am J Cardiol 2015;115(7):942–9.
5. Nombela-Franco L, Hélène E, Zahn R, et al. Clinical impact and evolution of mitral regurgitation following transcatheter aortic valve replacement: a meta-analysis. Heart 2015;101(17):1395–405.
6. Iung B, Baron G, Butchart EG, et al. A prospective survey of patients with valvular heart disease in Europe: the Euro Heart Survey on Valvular Heart Disease. Eur Heart J 2003;24(13):1231–43.
7. Barbanti M, Webb JG, Hahn RT, et al. Impact of preoperative moderate/severe mitral regurgitation on 2-year outcome after transcatheter and surgical aortic valve replacement. Circulation 2013;128(25):2776–84.
8. Sannino A, Losi MA, Schiattarella GG, et al. Meta-analysis of mortality outcomes and mitral regurgitation evolution in 4,839 patients having transcatheter aortic valve implantation for severe aortic stenosis. Am J Cardiol 2014;114(6):875–82.
9. Khan F, Okuno T, Malebranche D, et al. Transcatheter aortic valve replacement in patients with multivalvular heart disease. JACC Cardiovasc Interv 2020;13(13):1503–14.
10. Unger P, Pibarot P, Tribouilloy C, et al. Multiple and mixed valvular heart diseases. Circulation: Cardiovascular Imaging 2018;11(8):e007862.
11. Leavitt BJ, Baribeau YR, DiScipio AW, et al. Outcomes of patients undergoing concomitant aortic and mitral valve surgery in Northern New England. Circulation 2009;120(11_suppl_1):S155–62.
12. Otto CM, Nishimura RA, Bonow RO, et al. 2020 ACC/AHA guideline for the management of patients with valvular heart disease: a report of the American College of Cardiology/American Heart Association joint committee on clinical practice guidelines. Circulation 2021;143(5): e35–71.
13. Vahanian A, Beyersdorf F, Praz F, et al. 2021 ESC/EACTS guidelines for the management of valvular heart disease. Eur Heart J 2021;43(7):561–632.
14. Witberg G, Codner P, Landes U, et al. Effect of transcatheter aortic valve replacement on concomitant mitral regurgitation and its impact on mortality. JACC Cardiovasc Interv 2021;14(11): 1181–92.
15. Doldi PM, Steffen J, Stolz L, et al. Impact of mitral regurgitation aetiology on the outcomes of transcatheter aortic valve implantation. EuroIntervention 2023;19(6):526–36.
16. Bedogni F, Latib Azeem, De Marco Federico, et al. Interplay between mitral regurgitation and transcatheter aortic valve replacement with the corevalve revalving system. Circulation 2013;128(19): 2145–53.
17. Toggweiler S, Boone RH, Rodés-Cabau Josep, et al. Transcatheter aortic valve replacement. J Am Coll Cardiol 2012;59(23):2068–74.
18. Tzikas Apostolos, Piazza N, Dalen van, et al. Changes in mitral regurgitation after transcatheter aortic valve implantation. Cathet Cardiovasc Interv 2010;75(1):43–9. Published online January 1.
19. Hekimian G, Detaint D, Messika-Zeitoun D, et al. Mitral regurgitation in patients referred for transcatheter aortic valve implantation using the Edwards Sapien prosthesis: mechanisms and early postprocedural changes. J Am Soc Echocardiogr 2012;25(2):160–5.
20. Durst R, Avelar E, McCarty D, et al. Outcome and improvement predictors of mitral regurgitation after transcatheter aortic valve implantation. PubMed 2011;20(3):272–81.

21. Zahid S, Khalouf A, Hashem A, et al. Safety and feasibility of staged versus concomitant transcatheter edge-to-edge mitral valve repair after transcatheter aortic valve implantation. Am J Cardiol 2023;192:109–15.

22. Rudolph V, Schirmer J, Franzen O, et al. Bivalvular transcatheter treatment of high-surgical-risk patients with coexisting severe aortic stenosis and significant mitral regurgitation. Int J Cardiol 2013; 167(3):716–20.

23. Witberg G, Codner P, Landes U, et al. Transcatheter treatment of residual significant mitral regurgitation following TAVR: a multicenter registry. JACC Cardiovasc Interv 2020;13(23):2782–91.

24. Reid CL, Anton-Culver H, Yunis C, et al. Prevalence and clinical correlates of isolated mitral, isolated aortic regurgitation, and both in adults aged 21 to 35 years (from the CARDIA Study). Am J Cardiol 2007;99(6):830–4.

25. Singh JP, Evans JC, Levy D, et al. Prevalence and clinical determinants of mitral, tricuspid, and aortic regurgitation (the Framingham Heart Study). Am J Cardiol 1999;83(6):897–902.

26. Pai RG, Varadarajan P. Prognostic implications of mitral regurgitation in patients with severe aortic regurgitation. Circulation 2010;122(11_suppl_1):S43–7.

27. Aluru JS, Barsouk A, Saginala K, et al. Valvular heart disease epidemiology. Medical Sciences 2022; 10(2):32.

28. Unger P, Lancellotti P, Amzulescu M, et al. Pathophysiology and management of combined aortic and mitral regurgitation. Archives of Cardiovascular Diseases 2019;112(6–7):430–40.

29. Lim JY, Jung SH, Kim JB, et al. Management of concomitant mild to moderate functional mitral regurgitation during aortic valve surgery for severe aortic insufficiency. J Thorac Cardiovasc Surg 2014; 148(2):441–6.

30. Oettinger V, Hilgendorf I, Wolf D, et al. Treatment of pure aortic regurgitation using surgical or transcatheter aortic valve replacement between 2018 and 2020 in Germany. Frontiers in Cardiovascular Medicine 2023;10:1091983.

31. Zheng HJ, Cheng YB, Yan CJ, et al. Transfemoral transcatheter aortic valve replacement for pure native aortic regurgitation: one-year outcomes of a single-center study. BMC Cardiovasc Disord 2023;23(1):330.

32. Yokoyama H, Tamm AR, Geyer M, et al. Treatment of severe aortic valve regurgitation with the Trilogy TAVI system. EuroIntervention 2023;18(17):1444–5.

33. The JenaValve ALIGN-AR Pivotal Trial (ALIGN-AR). clinicaltrials.gov. Accessed August 13, 2023. https://clinicaltrials.gov/study/NCT04415047.

34. Aydin U, Gul M, Aslan S, et al. Concomitant transapical transcatheter valve implantations: Edwards Sapien valve for severe mitral regurgitation in a patient with failing mitral bioprostheses and JenaValve for the treatment of pure aortic regurgitation. Heart Surg Forum 2015;18(2):053.

35. Gerosa G, D'Onofrio A, Manzan E, et al. One-stage off-pump transapical mitral valve repair and aortic valve replacement. Circulation 2015;131(19):e430–4.

36. Pagnotta P, Sanz-Sánchez J, Regazzoli Damiano R, et al. One-stop-shop totally percutaneous approach for severe aortic and mitral regurgitation in cardiogenic shock. Cathet Cardiovasc Interv 2019;95(3):411–3.

37. Guerreiro C, Barbosa AR, Almeida J, et al. Sequential percutaneous approach for severe mitral and aortic regurgitation. Cureus 2020;12(1):e6619.

38. Bartko PE, Arfsten H, Frey MK, et al. Natural history of functional tricuspid regurgitation: implications of quantitative Doppler assessment. JACC (J Am Coll Cardiol): Cardiovascular Imaging 2019;12(3): 389–97.

39. Stone GW, Lindenfeld J, Abraham WT, et al. Transcatheter mitral-valve repair in patients with heart failure. N Engl J Med 2018;379(24):2307–18.

40. Topilsky Y, Maltais S, Medina Inojosa J, et al. Burden of tricuspid regurgitation in patients diagnosed in the community setting. JACC (J Am Coll Cardiol): Cardiovascular Imaging 2019;12(3): 433–42.

41. Reddy YNV, Obokata M, Verbrugge FH, et al. Atrial dysfunction in patients with heart failure with preserved ejection fraction and atrial fibrillation. J Am Coll Cardiol 2020;76(9):1051–64.

42. Shiran A, Sagie A. Tricuspid regurgitation in mitral valve disease incidence, prognostic implications, mechanism, and management. J Am Coll Cardiol 2009;53(5):401–8.

43. Muraru Denisa, Addetia K, Guta AC, et al. Right atrial volume is a major determinant of tricuspid annulus area in functional tricuspid regurgitation: a three-dimensional echocardiographic study. European Heart Journal Cardiovascular Imaging 2020;22(6):660–9.

44. Carpentier A, Deloche A, Hanania G, et al. Surgical management of acquired tricuspid valve disease. J Thorac Cardiovasc Surg 1974;67(1):53–65.

45. Blusztein DI, Hahn RT. New therapeutic approach for tricuspid regurgitation: transcatheter tricuspid valve replacement or repair. Frontiers in Cardiovascular Medicine 2023;10:1080101.

46. Taramasso M, Benfari G, van der Bijl P, et al. Transcatheter versus medical treatment of patients with symptomatic severe tricuspid regurgitation. J Am Coll Cardiol 2019;74(24):2998–3008.

47. Sannino A, Ilardi F, Hahn RT, et al. Clinical and echocardiographic outcomes of transcatheter tricuspid valve interventions: a systematic review and meta-analysis. Frontiers in Cardiovascular Medicine 2022;9:919395.

48. Sorajja P, Whisenant B, Hamid N, et al. Transcatheter repair for patients with tricuspid regurgitation.

N Engl J Med 2023;388(20):1833–42. Published online March 4.

49. Kodali SK, Hahn RT, Davidson CJ, et al. 1-year outcomes of transcatheter tricuspid valve repair. J Am Coll Cardiol 2023;81(18):1766–76.

50. Kodali S, Hahn RT, George I, et al. Transfemoral tricuspid valve replacement in patients with tricuspid regurgitation: TRISCEND study 30-day results. JACC Cardiovasc Interv 2022;15(5):471–80.

51. Webb JG, Chuang A, Meier D, et al. Transcatheter tricuspid valve replacement with the EVOQUE system. JACC Cardiovasc Interv 2022;15(5):481–91.

52. Georg Nickenig, Weber M, Schüler R, et al. Tricuspid valve repair with the Cardioband system: two-year outcomes of the multicentre, prospective TRI-REPAIR study. Eurointervention 2021;16(15):e1264–71.

53. Toyama K, Ayabe K, Kar S, et al. Postprocedural changes of tricuspid regurgitation after mitraclip therapy for mitral regurgitation. Am J Cardiol 2017;120(5):857–61.

54. Geyer M, Keller K, Bachmann K, et al. Concomitant tricuspid regurgitation severity and its secondary reduction determine long-term prognosis after transcatheter mitral valve edge-to-edge repair. Clin Res Cardiol 2021;110(5):676–88.

55. Kavsur R, Iliadis C, Spieker M, et al. Predictors and prognostic relevance of tricuspid alterations in patients undergoing transcatheter edge-to-edge mitral valve repair. EuroIntervention 2021;17(10):827–34.

56. Hahn RT, Asch FM, Weissman NJ, et al. Impact of tricuspid regurgitation on clinical outcomes. J Am Coll Cardiol 2020;76(11):1305–14.

57. Frangieh AH, Gruner C, Mikulicic F, et al. Impact of percutaneous mitral valve repair using the MitraClip system on tricuspid regurgitation. EuroIntervention 2016;11(14):E1680–6.

58. Sisinni A, Taramasso M, Praz F, et al. Concomitant transcatheter edge-to-edge treatment of secondary tricuspid and mitral regurgitation. An Expert Opinion. JACC: Cardiovascular Interventions 2023;16(2):127–39.

59. Meijerink F, Koch KT, Winter, et al. Tricuspid regurgitation after transcatheter mitral valve repair: clinical course and impact on outcome. Cathet Cardiovasc Interv 2021;98(3):E427–35.

60. Mehr M, Karam N, Taramasso Maurizio, et al. Combined tricuspid and mitral versus isolated mitral valve repair for severe MR and TR.

61. Stocker TF, Hertell H, Orban M, et al. Cardiopulmonary hemodynamic profile predicts mortality after transcatheter tricuspid valve repair in chronic heart failure. JACC Cardiovasc Interv 2021;14(1):29–38.

62. Brener MI, Lurz P, Hausleiter J, et al. Right ventricular-pulmonary arterial coupling and afterload reserve in patients undergoing transcatheter tricuspid valve repair. J Am Coll Cardiol 2022;79(5):448–61.

63. Shih E, George TJ, DiMaio JM, et al. Contemporary outcomes of isolated tricuspid valve surgery. J Surg Res 2023;283:1–8.

64. Varma P, Krishna N, Jose R, et al. Ischemic mitral regurgitation. Ann Card Anaesth 2017;20(4):432.

65. Aklog L, Filsoufi F, Flores KQ, et al. Does coronary artery bypass grafting alone correct moderate ischemic mitral regurgitation? Circulation 2001;104(12 Suppl 1):I68–75.

66. Bax JJ, Braun J, Somer ST, et al. Restrictive annuloplasty and coronary revascularization in ischemic mitral regurgitation results in reverse left ventricular remodeling. Circulation 2004;110(11_suppl_1):II103–8.

67. Ec M, Am G, Eh B, et al. Recurrent mitral regurgitation after annuloplasty for functional ischemic mitral regurgitation. J Thorac Cardiovasc Surg 2004;128(6):916–24.

68. Hung J, Papakostas Lampros, Tahta SA, et al. Mechanism of recurrent ischemic mitral regurgitation after annuloplasty. Circulation 2004;110(11_suppl_1):II85–90.

69. Obadia JF, Messika-Zeitoun D, Leurent G, et al. Percutaneous repair or medical treatment for secondary mitral regurgitation. N Engl J Med 2018;379(24):2297–306.

70. Stone GW, Abraham WT, Lindenfeld J, et al. Five-year follow-up after transcatheter repair of secondary mitral regurgitation. N Engl J Med 2023;388:2037–48.

71. Hausleiter J, Stocker TJ, Adamo M, Karam N, Swaans MJ, Praz F. Mitral valve transcatheter edge-to-edge repair. EuroIntervention. Published 2023. https://eurointervention.pcronline.com/article/mitral-valve-transcatheter-edge-to-edge-repair.

72. Lim DS, Herrmann HC, Grayburn P, et al. Consensus document on non-suitability for transcatheter mitral valve repair by edge-to-edge therapy. Structural Heart 2021;5(3):227–33.

Moving?

Make sure your subscription moves with you!

To notify us of your new address, find your **Clinics Account Number** (located on your mailing label above your name), and contact customer service at:

Email: journalscustomerservice-usa@elsevier.com

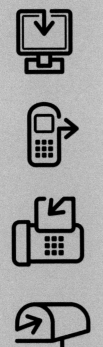

800-654-2452 (subscribers in the U.S. & Canada)
314-447-8871 (subscribers outside of the U.S. & Canada)

Fax number: 314-447-8029

Elsevier Health Sciences Division
Subscription Customer Service
3251 Riverport Lane
Maryland Heights, MO 63043

ELSEVIER